1001

Questions to Ask
Before Having a Baby

ALSO BY MONICA MENDEZ LEAHY

1001 Questions to Ask Before You Get Married

1001

QUESTIONS TO ASK
BEFORE HAVING A BABY

Monica Mendez Leahy

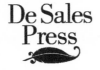

De Sales
Press

De Sales Press
106.5 Judge J. Aiso Street #266
Los Angeles, CA 90012
www.desalespress.com

Ordering Information:
Special discounts are available on quantity purchases by corporations, associations, and others. For details, contact the publisher at the address above.

Printed in the United States of America

First Edition

13 14 15 16 17 18 19 20 / 10 9 8 7 6 5 4 3 2 1

Publisher's Cataloging-in-Publication Data

Leahy, Monica Mendez.
    1001 questions to ask before having a baby / Monica Mendez Leahy.
    p. cm.
    ISBN- 9780989567701

1. Pregnancy. 2. Childbirth. 3. Postnatal care. 4. Parenting. 5. Parenthood. I. One thousand and one questions to ask before having a baby. II. Title.

RG525 .L38 2013
618.24 --dc23
2013943677

Edited by Context Editorial Services

Cover design by La Shea V. Ortiz

Interior design by NuImage Design

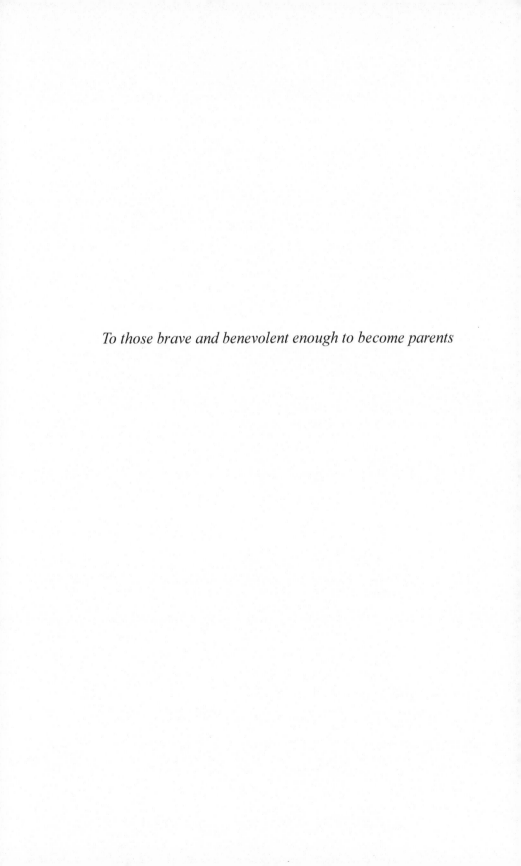

To those brave and benevolent enough to become parents

CONTENTS

Chapter 6

Chapter 7

Chapter 8

Chapter 9

INTRODUCTION

When the first draft of this book was finished, there were over 3,000 questions. I thought inquiries such as "How long do you expect your mother to stay and help you with the baby?" and "Will you keep blogging about your child even if she asked you to stop?" were important enough to list. But alas, the title of this book forced me to take an ax in hand for some serious chopping.

I bring up this heavy editing as a disclaimer that, although there are over 1,000 questions to consider before having a baby in this book, some readers may wonder why there aren't more questions regarding social media, estate planning, childhood obesity, or college savings plans. Here's the answer: If the initial 1,000 plus questions act as a catalyst for future parents to discuss how they will approach these under-addressed subjects plus several more, then the book has done its job. Broad in scope as this book may be, it's only a kick-off to a lifetime of questions parents will ask themselves over and over again as they search for the elusive answers for how best to raise their child.

This book aims to prepare, not scare, future parents for the duties and quandaries tied up with bringing a new life into the world. Destiny may have already paved the road your family will travel, but ultimately, you're in the driver's seat. The questions in this book will give you an idea what types of forks and detours you're likely to encounter down the road, and allow you to contemplate how to maneuver through these twists and turns on the path ahead. There is no greater responsibility than to care for someone completely reliant on you for guidance, and the risk of going down the parenthood highway without a roadmap too perilous.

CHAPTER 1

A Baby Changes Everything

What changes should you expect after having a baby?

*"The hardest thing to do after having my children was to let go. I'm a Type A personality, and if I expected everything to always be perfect, I would drive myself and probably my own kids crazy. I had to surrender to the chaos. And you know, it was OK. I just had to...*surrender.*"*

-Tina, mother of four boys ages 4 to 14 years old

"A baby changes everything;" at least that's what everyone keeps telling you. Aside from the lack of sleep, endless laundry, and trading in the two-seater for a minivan, what other changes can you expect? To gauge the accuracy of your vision of life post-delivery (or adoption), finish each sentence below with the statement that best describes how you see your future as the uber-cool parent you expect to be. You might find it interesting to re-visit your answers in a year or two, and see if they were clairvoyant or amusingly clueless.

After the baby arrives...

1) you'll shop for shoes and think,

    a) "These red patent stilettos are hot!"

    b) "These Clarks are kind of cute!"

2) falling asleep on the sofa before 7:30 p.m. will be...

    a) something grandparents do.

    b) a daily occurrence.

3) bodily functions such as your baby's taking a poo or pee will be...

    a) discussed in private.

    b) ~~blogged~~ about incessantly.

c laughed about

4) you'll be grossed out by...

    a) funky body odors, puke, head lice.

    b) nothing, really.

c all of it

5) you'll usually introduce yourself as... *audience*

    a) Ms. or Mrs. So-and-So.

    b) ~~Joey's~~ mom.

6) you'll dream about...

    a) winning the lottery.

    b) taking a long shower sometime during daylight hours.

7) you'll be amazed at how much you can accomplish...

    a) in just one day.

    b) with just one hand and a baby on your hip.

8) by midafternoon you'll need...

    a) two cups of coffee to get going.

    b) ~~two glasses of wine to keep going.~~

9) you'll view your breasts as...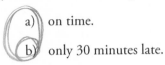

    a) erogenous zones.

    b) a nutritional destination.

10) ~~your social media~~ page will be full of ...

    a) pictures of you in cute outfits.

    b) pictures of your baby in cute outfits.

11) you'll strive to arrive at places...

    a) on time.

    b) only 30 minutes late.

12) a moment of peace and quiet in your house will mean...

    a) you can relax for a few precious minutes.

    b) something or someone is up to no good.

13) when telemarketers call, you'll...

    a) hang up immediately.

    b) relish the opportunity to have an adult conversation.

14) the fashion goal you've set for yourself post-baby is to...

    a) be the cute mom in the cute outfits.

    b) not wear the same sweats and faded tee shirt more than five days in a row.

15) you purchase extra-large sunglasses...

    a) to look hip and protect your eyes while pushing a stroller outdoors.

    b) so nobody recognizes you without makeup and with bad hair while pushing a stroller outdoors.

16) when you cross a long bridge over a river, you'll...

    a)   feel lucky to share such a beautiful view with your new baby.

    b)   check everyone's seat belt, and envision various rescue and first aid maneuvers should you plunge into the water below.

17) when you meet a potential girlfriend you'll think...

    a)   I hope she's fun to hang around with.

    b)   I hope she's available to babysit.

18) you'll schedule "me time" to...

    a)   get a much-needed mani-pedi.

    b)   go to the bathroom uninterrupted.

19) you'll decide to train for your first marathon to...

    a)   get back in shape after the baby.

    b)   have at least one activity that is solitary and not baby related.

20) your favorite tee shirt will be ...

    a)   a tight little v-neck that makes you looks slim and sexy.

    b)   a patterned crew neck that hides spit-up.

21) you will schedule your days...

    a)   according to the clock.

    b)   according to naps.

22) you'll be tempted to walk around naked...

    a)   to show you're still sexy and hot to trot.

    b)   to have less laundry to do.

23) you'll use time-outs when...

    a)   your child has a tantrum or meltdown.

    b)   you're about to have a tantrum or meltdown.

24) the appliance you expect to use less is…

    a)   the clothes dryer.

    b)   your blow dryer.

25) you'll know all the words to…

    a)   your favorite hip-hop song.

    b)   the hip-hop fuzzy bunny song.

If you chose option "b" as your answer to the majority of the questions above, congratulations! Your mind is already in parental mode.

What makes a "Dude" a "Daddy"?

"I have to admit, it's the mother's time when she's pregnant. Yes, you're excited, but you don't really feel like it's real yet; maybe it's because the baby isn't inside you. But the moment the baby is born, it's a total transformation. You realize that any decision you make will directly affect another life—no, two other people's lives. You can't believe you've been given that kind of power. It's extremely empowering."

-Peter, father of a 1-month-old son

Becoming a dad doesn't mean your dreams of adventure and business success have to die. As a friend once questioned Peter Clemens, author of *thechangeblog. com*, "Why can't you have a baby and still travel the world and make money?" To which the surprising answer is, you can. Many fathers find they're *more* motivated to achieve their aspirations. They look forward to sharing the fruits of their success with their child, while being very aware of the type of path they'll lay down as they blaze a trail toward the future.

Will you change from a "dude" to a "daddy" state of mind? To find out, choose the answer that you think will best describe your feelings as a newly minted father.

After your baby is born...

1) your main motive in life will be...

  a) to make millions of dollars.

  b) to make your kid proud of you.

2) you'll say things like "I'll kill anyone who...

  a) scratches my new truck" –and be joking.

  b) lays a finger on my child"–and mean it.

3) house fires, choking on food, drowning, kidnapping are things...

  a) you read about or see on dramatic TV programs.

  b) you constantly fear will happen to your child.

4) you'll look back on your pre-baby life and think...

  a) those were the good ol' days.

  b) boy, was my life boring.

5) saving the whales, protecting our national parks, and demanding clean drinking water will be causes...

  a) you believe are for lefty wackos and tree huggers.

  b) you'll volunteer for to make the planet a better place for your baby.

6) an afternoon round of golf will mean…

    a) cursing on the green when you miss a put.

    b) giggling uncontrollably when you can't get the ball up the ramp and into the mini windmill.

7) spending Saturday afternoons hanging out with friends bragging about past exploits sounds like…

    a) a great idea, there's nothing else you'd rather do.

    b) a lame idea, there's so many other things you'd rather do.

8) you'll see a flashy motorcycle tear down your street and think…

    a) "That bike's sick! Where can I get one?"

    b) "That bike should slow down! Where's a cop when you need one?"

9) you'll catch a glimpse of your reflection while walking down the street and think…

    a) "I wonder if I'm still a chick magnet?"

    b) "Who knew this baby would be such a chick magnet?!"

10) you'll memorize the names of…

    a) all the players on the L.A. Lakers.

    b) all the characters on the Muppets.

11) fantasizing about a new set of wheels will mean…

    a) you're ready to get a new car.

    b) you're ready to invest in a new stroller.

12) you'll spend hours thinking of how to look cool…

    a) in front of women.

    b) in a minivan.

13) the best way to get over a bad day at work is to...

    a)   play poker and watch ESPN.

    b)   play peek-a-boo and watch the Disney Channel.

14) when you see the quarterback throw a winning touchdown at a Super Bowl, you'll think....

    a)   that should be me on the field.

    b)   one day that will be my kid on the field.

15) you'll feel like a superhero when you...

    a)   make your partner scream in bed.

    b)   make your baby stop screaming in your arms.

16) your motivation for getting back in shape will be to...

    a)   look better naked.

    b)   to keep up with your kid, who runs around naked.

17) your motto is to "Live...

    a)   for the day."

    b)   for the future."

18) your phone has a total of...

    a)   20 random photos taken throughout the past year.

    b)   200 baby pictures taken yesterday.

19) once your shift ends at work...

    a)   you'll hang around to share a few laughs with your co-workers.

    b)   you'll rush home to share a few laughs with your baby.

20) you'll swear that any man who...

    a)   changes a diaper is a wuss.

    b)   can't change a diaper is a wuss.

If you chose "b" as your answer to most the questions, you're well prepared for your future life in Daddyland.

How Will a Baby Change Your Relationship with Your Partner?

"Fortunately, my husband is a night owl, so he was in charge of the late night feedings. I couldn't wait to hit the bed! When we decided that our babies were ready to sleep in their own crib, my husband, the night owl, was in charge of watching the baby during the weaning period. Raising a child is straining—both in a good and bad way. First you're a couple, now you're a family. You're really happy—but the responsibilities! The relationship dynamic changes and you have to change with it. That's life; you just don't throw in the towel."

-Judy, mother of a 12-year-old daughter and a 17-year-old son

Having a threesome (you, your partner, and the baby) means beefing up your teamwork skills, which will constantly be put to the test. Don't expect a 50-50 percent division of labor; when has life ever been fair and equal? View your partnership like the thermostat in your home: the heater does all of the work during one season, while the air conditioner runs overtime during the other. Then there is the wacky year when the A/C seems to run all 12 months.

Working separately, answer the questions below. Choose the option that best describes your expectations. Once done, share your answers with your partner to better understand how you'll each respond to changes in your relationship, and to create a plan on how to cope with these changes.

1) Whose life is expected to change the most by the arrival of your baby?

    a) Mostly yours

    b) Mostly your partner's.

    c) Yours and your partner's equally.

2) How will you share responsibilities so that one person doesn't feel overwhelmed by the demands of caring for a newborn?

    a) Discuss and create a written schedule of assigned duties.

    b) Just try to help each other out whenever possible.

    c) Call for mom or hire Super Nanny.

3) How would you feel if your partner accused you of becoming too "baby obsessed"?

    a) I'd be a little hurt, but would try to change.

    b) I'd say, "Join my OCD club, I need another member."

    c) I'd feel she/he was just being needy, and should learn to cope.

4) Will you make sure you talk about things other than the baby with your partner?

    a) Nope, the baby should be the focus of our lives, 24/7.

    b) We'll try, but it will be very hard to do.

    c) Absolutely, we refuse to become parents that can ONLY talk about their kid.

5) How would you feel if your partner wanted to join a book group, bowling league, or poker club that required nights away from you and the baby?

    a) I would be livid. Being a parent means giving up personal hobbies.

    b) It wouldn't bother me at all.

    c) It's OK as long as I get a free afternoon of shopping for every afternoon he's away.

6) Whom would you turn to for advice if you felt your partner wasn't into caring for the baby as much as you would like?

    a) I would talk to friends or family members that have gone through a similar experience.

    b) I would get anonymous help online or with a counselor.

    c) I'd prefer to keep the problem "in house" and try to work it out as a couple.

7) How often will you insist on spending time alone and reconnecting as a couple?

    a) On special occasions like Valentine's Day or our anniversary.

    b) At least once a day, but never less than once a week.

    c) We can reconnect once the baby leaves for college.

8) What would be a sign that you're losing touch with your partner and need help or counseling?

    a) You're fighting more often, or you suspect postpartum depression is affecting your relationship.

    b) You're not fighting more, but spending less and less time together.

    c) You're beginning to have romantic feelings for someone other than your partner.

9) Will you let chores, your job, and baby activities take priority over your couple time?

    a) Yes. You just have to let some things go to make room for all the new responsibilities.

    b) Yes, it's more important to see my baby happy than to have a happy relationship with my partner.

    c) No way. Even if the Queen of England invited us over for dinner, our date night would be non-negotiable.

10) Which of the following would bother you the most?

    a)   Your partner showing ignorance in how to care for a baby.

    b)   Your partner showing a lack of interest in caring for baby.

    c)   Your partner relying too much on a parent for help with the baby.

11) What would you say if your partner accused you of neglecting his or her needs over the baby's?

    a)   "Get over it, you had your turn."

    b)   "Come over so mama/papa can give you a big hug too."

    c)   "What about MY needs, you selfish brat?"

12) Would you kick your partner out of bed to let your young child sleep with you?

    a)   Yes, I want to enjoy co-sleeping for as long as possible.

    b)   Only if our child had a terrible nightmare.

    c)   No. It's not fair to my partner, plus children have to learn to sleep in their own bed.

13) How will you cope if you completely lost your sexual desire for your partner after the birth of your baby?

    a)   Assume it's a phase that will end in a few months.

    b)   Freak out, comb the web for advice, and make an appointment to see a doctor.

    c)   Load up on the porn or romance novels in fear that the magic has gone out of your relationship.

14) Will you keep toys, videos, plastic play equipment or stuffed animals in your bedroom?

    a)   Yes, we want our child to feel free to play anywhere.

    b)   Only if there isn't room for the stuff elsewhere.

    c)   No. Our bedroom will be our adult-only sanctuary.

15) How would you like your partner to respond to your post-pregnancy body?

    a)   I want him to say I look beautiful even if I've gained 50 pounds.

    b)   I want him to encourage me to stick to a diet and exercise routine.

    c)   If he says one word, good or bad, about my muffin top, I'll crack his kneecaps.

There are no right or wrong answers to the previous questions, only opinions that couples have to work with and adjust as they strive for unity through compromise.

How will your relationships with your parents change after the birth of your baby?

"There's a club you join when you're a dad. You get a certain amount of respect once you have a baby. I don't know if it's pity or respect. I noticed a change in my in-laws. It felt like they looked at me and thought 'OK, now you're legit!'"

    -Scott, father of a 9-year-old daughter
    and 12- and 16-year-old sons

Conventional wisdom has it that whatever type of relationship you've had with your parents or in-laws before having a baby, it will be magnified once you bring your bundle-of-love home. If you get along superbly with mom and dad, you'll become even closer. If your in-laws are slightly annoying, they'll become intolerable. In addition to inflated sentiments, expectations can be completely out of whack. If you want to increase your chances of having a positive relationship (or defy wisdom by improving a shaky one) with your parents and in-laws, you'll want to plan a course of action on the common gripes against grandparents touched upon below.

Choose a solution to the following hypothetical questions. If a question specifically mentions mothers, go back and answer it a second time, asking yourself if your answer would be different if "mother" were replaced with "mother-in-law," "father," or "father-in-law."

What would you do if...

1) you appreciated their help, but your parent's every move or word is starting to drive you crazy?

    a) Cry in your room alone and feel guilty about your feelings.

    b) Tell them you love them, but are feeling a little anxious and need some space.

    c) Be direct and blurt out, "You're driving me crazy. Back off!"

2) your mother started taking over your parenting duties?

    a) Convince yourself that her dominance is better (and cheaper) than hiring a full-time nanny.

    b) Work together to set house rules; assign yourselves specific tasks and boundaries.

    c) Gently but firmly say it's your turn to be a mother; her time is over.

3) your mother showed little interest in spending time with your baby or refused to babysit?

   a) Feel hurt by her selfishness and avoid spending time with her when possible.

   b) I would delicately bring it up and try to understand her reasons without being judgmental.

   c) Ask why she bothered having any children if she had no desire to become a grandmother.

4) your mother kept bringing over gifts of toys and clothes that your child really doesn't need or want?

   a) Roll your eyes when she brings a package, and then sell the gift at your next yard sale.

   b) Explain that you appreciate the gesture, but future gifts will be donated to charity.

   c) Scold her for "wasting" her money and not following your rules.

5) your mother paid more attention to her other grandkids than your own child?

   a) Retaliate by spending more time with your mother-in-law and playing up all the fun you're having together.

   b) Think it was her loss, and go about your life as normal.

   c) Insist you won't tolerate her playing favorites like she did when you were a child.

6) your mother posted pictures of your naked toddler on her social media page?

   a) You wouldn't like it, but you'd let this crazy grandma behavior slide.

   b) Nothing; your child is so cute, how could she resist?

   c) Freak out and threaten to post naked pictures of her online if they aren't removed.

7) your mother invited people over to see the baby without asking you first?

    a)   Cringe and bear it to keep the peace.

    b)   Explain that the baby is sleeping and can't be disturbed, but you're happy to arrange another time for a visit.

    c)   Complain to your partner and have him/her fix the problem.

8) you constantly heard your mother complain that she never sees the baby, is sent pictures, or is allowed to take the baby out alone?

    a)   Block her calls, lock the doors, and take a break from seeing her for a month or more.

    b)   Calmly explain that because her complaints stress you out, you'll be limiting the amount of time you'll spend together unless she changes her tone.

    c)   Say, "Talk to the hand, Grandma!"

9) your mother kept commenting on your every parenting decision during visits?

    a)   Ignore her comments; she's just trying to feel important.

    b)   Firmly say, "My baby, my rules," and walk away with your baby.

    c)   Confront her and say, "Diss me once more, and you'll never see your grandkid again!"

10) having your mother stay to help with your baby has given you *more* work, not less?

    a)   Drop hints that suggest you can manage without her.

    b)   Explain that you appreciated her help, but now you're insisting she go home and you'll call her when needed.

    c)   While crying, let her know that she's been more work than the baby has, and you can't take it any longer.

If you mostly chose option "a," you prefer to suffer and simmer in silence. This may keep all quiet on the home front, but you run the risk of blowing up when the stress and your postpartum hormones bubble over. If option b) was your most frequent choice, you have the diplomatic skills of a good parent–and U.N. member. If option c) tops your list, you may believe honesty is the best policy, but you seem to deliver it via sledgehammer. Hard as it may be to bite your tongue when each of your actions is followed up with an unsolicited comment on how you can do better, successfully dealing with anyone, in-laws or your partner, requires choosing your battles wisely. When you feel you must speak up, kindly remind your parents that they had their chance to make mistakes, now it's yours.

Do you expect your pre-baby friends to stick around?

"She's still my friend, and all, but when I visit her, only half listens to me because she's always looking over at her kid. Our conversations are always interrupted because she's yelling, 'Suzie, don't touch that! Suzie, sit down! Suzie, don't do that!' Her kid is cute, I guess, but I mean, do you think it would be rude if I didn't call her until she (the child) was, like, 18?"

-Overheard café discussion in Los Angeles

Honest discussions with your friends are a good way to gauge which ones will stick with you during the diaper years and beyond, but more crucial is the conversation you should have with yourself. What are you expecting from your friends once you go from childfree to child-bound?

Hurt feelings and misunderstandings between friends are often the result of unmet expectations.

Answer the questions below, and then discuss your responses with your closest friend. Choose someone who will tell you straight if you're demanding too much from others who, although they love you, may need a bit more time to adjust to a child-rearing environment.

Are you expecting your friends to...

1. share in your excitement about expecting a baby?
2. pitch in and help you acquire nursery items?
3. visit you regularly once your baby has been born?
4. invite you to the same parties or hangouts you attended before having a baby?
5. hang out at your house the same amount of time as before you had a baby?
6. never scold your child, even if he does something naughty?
7. help watch your child while you take a shower or run an errand?
8. buy your child birthday or Christmas/Chanukah gifts?
9. ask to see baby pictures or get updates about his development?
10. keep you company while you watch your child play at a park or playground?

If several of your current friends already have families of their own, the conversion from being a childless friend to a member of the parenthood club may be a welcomed change. Be the first one of your clique to produce offspring, however, and the transition may not be so smooth. That's not to say you'll lose all your pre-baby friends within your first trimester. Friendships naturally wax and wane, and a friend that may back off during your child's infant years could come back to be your biggest supporter during your child's terrible twos.

Gerald, the father of two school-age daughters, was happy to see that parenthood had little effect on his pre-baby social group. "My friendships with people who didn't have kids didn't really change," he recalls. "I got closer to the friends that had babies around the same time as I did, because we could relate. The ones that had older kids, they just gave me a look every now and then, and while nodding would say, 'Now it's your turn!'"

How will your four-legged or feathered friends react to a new baby?

"The less your baby reaches out to touch your dog, the more comfortable your dog will feel around your baby. The more comfortable your dog feels, the safer it is for your baby."

> -Madeline Gabriel, creator of the
> "Dogs and Babies Play it Safe" training program

Professional trainer of pets and pet owners Madeline Gabriel believes a big mistake parents make is insisting their baby and pet become playmates. "Your dog belongs to you, not the baby, nor the baby to the dog." This erroneous desire for physical camaraderie may be one reason why the Journal of Injury Prevention found dogs that bite children most often have never before bitten a child. Proof that even the most laid-back pet can suddenly start showing signs of aggression toward a child. The best scenario between baby and pet, according to Gabriel, is "mutual indifference."

Let's see if you can choose the best answer to the questions below on how to ensure peace and harmony between fur, feathers, scales, and a new baby.

1) Which of the following are good techniques for preparing a pet for your baby's arrival?

   a) Walk your dog while pushing a stroller.

   b) Teach your pet alternative behaviors like lying next to, not jumping on, furniture.

   c) Have your pet regularly see you do daily tasks around the house while holding a bundle.

   d) All of the above.

2) What's the best way to introduce your newborn to a pet?

   a) Put your newborn up to the animal's face and say, "Here's your new friend."

   b) Put your baby on the floor and let the pet sniff and lick his/her face.

   c) Give your pet a treat while holding the baby to create good will.

   d) Only let your pet sniff your baby while in your arms, and only if the pet shows an interest. Then get up and walk away without speaking.

3) What should you do if your baby develops a magnetic attraction to cats or dogs?

   a) Encourage his love of animals by showing him how to gently pet the animal.

   b) Have him play with the cat or dog as much as possible so they bond.

    c)   Keep your cat or dog outside and out of view.

    d)   Distract your child with toys while teaching him that the animals are best observed, not touched.

4) What common pet items should not be within touching distance of a crawling baby or toddler?

    a)   Aquariums or birdcages.

    b)   Food and water bowls.

    c)   Litter boxes.

    d)   All of the above.

5) What are some pets that the American Academy of Pediatrics does NOT recommend for children under five years of age?

    a)   Reptiles (turtles, snakes, lizards, iguanas).

    b)   Rodents (hamsters, guinea pigs, rats, chinchillas).

    c)   Musteloidea (ferrets, skunks, minks).

    d)   All of the above.

6) What changes would force you to consider giving away your beloved pet?

    a)   Growling and snapping at your child or anyone that comes near your child.

    b)   Destructive behavior (urinating on rugs, chewing or ripping up furniture).

    c)   Constant barking or whining for attention.

    d)   None of the above. I would rather spend a small fortune on animal trainers than give up my beloved pet.

The correct answer for questions 1-5 is "d." Any of the answers for question number 6 can be correct as long your decision can guarantee your child's safety. Anyone who has grown up with a family pet knows the love and lasting warm memories they can bring. However, never let your love for a pet, or animals in general, impair your judgment and trick you into having a false sense of security when they are around your child. Nobody responds well to a forced friendship. When that friendship involves an animal and a toddler, it could be downright dangerous.

What changes should you expect back in the office?

"I'm very career driven, so before he was born I wondered, 'Will I be able to let go?' But now, and my co-workers know this, when it's time to leave work, I go. I know that in the end, your family will be there, not your job."

-Carmine, father of a 17-month-old son

Some women dread going back to the office after the birth of their child. Others welcome it impatiently. Working for a company with child-friendly policies and a pro-family culture certainly makes juggling your parenting and professional demands easier. But what will you do if you have to work with an unsympathetic boss who is annoyed by your request for breast-pumping breaks? Or if your mind keeps wandering back to your baby and you just can't concentrate on your work?

The questions below address some of the changes you may encounter in your work environment —or your attitude—before and after delivering your baby. Choose the answer that best reflects your expectations and likely behavior as a working parent.

1) What changes are you expecting at work when you return from maternity leave?

   a) None, it will be the same old grind.

   b) More flexible hours and longer breaks to check on the baby and pump milk.

2) What would you do if nobody in the office asked to see a picture of your baby or asked how your baby is doing?

   a) You wouldn't be surprised. It's all about the job, not personal endeavors.

   b) You would be hurt. You thought your co-workers were your friends.

3) What would you do if you felt your co-workers resented you for leaving early or taking extra days off to care for your child?

   a) Ignore their negative attitude and just do your job.

   b) Discuss their bad attitudes with your boss and ask that they be supportive of motherhood.

4) Will you frequently talk about your baby and put up lots of baby pictures around your work area?

   a) No. As always, you'll keep your personal life separate – at home, not at work.

   b) Yes; how could anyone keep quiet about something as precious as a little baby?

5) If you were not assigned a certain project, or were passed over for a promotion, would you automatically think it was just because you decided to have a baby?

    a) No. You're confident your company did not factor in pregnancy when making their decision.

    b) Yes. Companies usually don't like to promote young mothers.

If you mostly chose option "a," you're expecting it to be business as usual in the office when you return from maternity leave. However, don't short-change yourself by assuming nothing has changed. You now may qualify for generous family leave policies or maternity allowances allowed by your employer. Find out what provisions your company offers, and don't be afraid to take advantage of them.

If you mostly chose option "b," you may be expecting too many changes in your office. Yes, you have just given birth to or adopted a little miracle that you want to show off to the world, but everyone has work to do. Don't let your delight in sharing your experiences turn into an office distraction. Motherhood does not give you an excuse to slack off.

How much does it cost to care for a child?

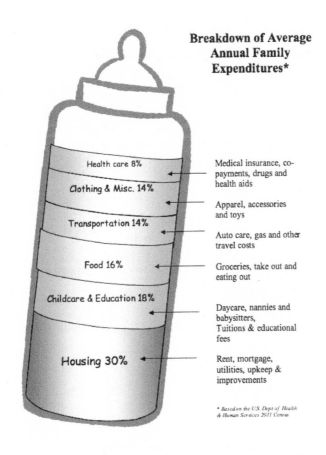

**Breakdown of Average
Annual Family
Expenditures***

Health care 8% — Medical insurance, co-payments, drugs and health aids

Clothing & Misc. 14% — Apparel, accessories and toys

Transportation 14% — Auto care, gas and other travel costs

Food 16% — Groceries, take out and eating out

Childcare & Education 18% — Daycare, nannies and babysitters, Tuitions & educational fees

Housing 30% — Rent, mortgage, utilities, upkeep & improvements

* Based on the U.S. Dept of Health & Human Services 2011 Census

How much will you spend to create a comfortable and baby-safe home?

"When my baby was born I kept her in the closet...literally. We lived with my mother at the time, and all my husband and I had was one room. I fixed up the closet, which had no doors, and was the perfect size for a bassinette. It was fine. It worked. How much room does a baby really need?"

-Belinda, mother of a 22-year-old daughter and 19-year-old son

Living with your in-laws or parents rent-free is a great money-saver, but it's usually a temporary arrangement. Most couples with children eventually move into homes of their own and take on the most expensive living expense: housing. Paying for, furnishing, and keeping a home comfortable will be your biggest expense, taking up anywhere from 30-32 percent of your household expenditures.

Below is a list of housing projects and purchases commonly taken on by first-time parents. Before you whip out that credit card, ask yourself if the expense is necessary and affordable. However, never, ever choose savings over safety. Choosing an inexpensive apartment with a door that opens up to a busy highway or a free crib that's been recalled due to defects is dangerous, not a deal.

How will having a baby change your home surroundings?	Enter "Yes" or "No"	Estimated $ Cost (+) or Savings (-)
Will you be …		
moving to a larger home after the birth of your child?	maybe	_____
moving in with relatives to save money?	No	_____
adding or renovating any rooms to accommodate your new baby?	maybe	_____
hiring a housecleaner, gardener, or handy man for home maintenance help?	maybe	_____
spending more on utilities to run appliances and heat/cool your home?	?	_____
upgrade your TV, Internet or phone service?	no	_____
putting items into a paid storage facility to make room for a nursery?	yes	_____
buying any appliances, such a bigger clothes washer and dryer?	no	_____
moving to a family-friendly community with better schools, cultural amenities, and childhood programs?	no	_____
asking a roommate who shares expenses to move out?	n/a	_____

	Enter "Yes" or "No"	Estimated $ Cost (+) or Savings (-)
Will you be buying a...		
crib or bassinette and bedding?	_yes_	_____
changing table?	_yes ?._	_____
dresser drawers?	_____	_____
rocking chair?	_yes_	_____
toy chest?	_____	_____
toddler bed?	_____	_____
child-sized table and chair?	_____	_____
play yard?	_____	_____
high chair or booster seat?	_____	_____
bookcase or storage shelves?	_____	_____

Which of the following will you do to childproof your home?	Enter "Yes" or "No"	Estimated $ Cost (+) or Savings (-)
Remove any thorny or toxic plants from your yard?	_____	_____
Install a fence or gate around a pool, or to separate animals or enclose your property?	_____	_____
Drain a pool, fountain, or pond?	_____	_____

Which of the following will you do to childproof your home?	**Enter "Yes" or "No"**	**Estimated $ Cost (+) or Savings (-)**
Install locks or nail shut an entrance to crawl spaces, doggy doors, or outdoor shed?		
Get rid of old appliances or machinery stored outside?		
Discard any animal traps?		
Buy a lockable cabinet or storage house to hold tools, chemicals, weapons, and other dangerous items?	yes	
Install security screens or locks on windows or doors leading outside?	yes	
Bolt down televisions, bookcases, lamps, or tabletop decorations that can be tipped over?	yes	
Remove floor-length drapes, and make sure shade pulls and short drapes are not within a toddler's reach?		
Install a fireplace screen or radiator cover and remove any matches, pokers, or andirons?	yes	
Install safety locks on all drawers, cabinet doors, and toilets?	yes	
Unplug and put away electric razors, hair dryers, or other electronic gadgets while not in use?		
Replace any glass items such as cups, soap dispensers, or decorations with items made out of plastic?		
Remove a bathroom wall heater?		
Remove any ceiling fans?		

Which of the following will you do to childproof your home?	Enter "Yes" or "No"	Estimated $ Cost (+) or Savings (-)
Put guardrails on any bed your baby may sleep on?		
Remove any locks on doors that only lock from the inside?		
Trim back any large tree branches reachable from bedroom windows?		
Install smoke and carbon monoxide detectors?		
Refit stair banister balusters that have gaps of more than 4" wide?		
Install safety latches or knob covers on appliances and faucet handles?		
Install outlet covers and safety locks on electrical switchboxes?		
Put up a safety gate at the top of the staircase or in doorways?		
Move furniture away from edge of a balcony, window, or counter?		

Making your home child-safe may add a pretty penny to your already high housing costs, but when you learn that half of all childhood deaths are from accidental injuries such as falls, drowning, or suffocation, and every three weeks* a child dies from a TV tip-over**, the costs may seem immaterial.

*U.S. Centers for Disease Control and Prevention (Vital Signs 2013).

** Safe Kids Worldwide (Did You Know? 2013).

How much will you spend on child care?

"I worked as a nanny and was gone for 12 hours the first day I returned to work. I decided that staying home with my own son was the way to go. Sadly that means my husband works 80+ hours a week. At first I thought I was being selfish but my husband explained to me that it was a sacrifice we were all making for our son."

-Brigitte, stay-at-home-parent

You've probably heard of college savings plans, but should you start investing to be able to afford child care if needed? A report by ChildCare Aware, the largest child care resource and referral agency, states that the cost of day care in many cities can surpass the yearly tuition of an in-state university, which leads many parents to question if working to pay for day care makes financial sense. Using the U.S. Department of Health & Human Services statistic that 17 percent of a family's budget is spent on child care and education is too general to accurately calculate what you will be paying for these services. Your percentage will depend on the day care choices you make (covered in more detail in Chapter 7) and the options available in your area.

Can you afford to be a SAHP?

Having a stay-at-home-parent (SAHP) is the ultimate dream for many families and a possibility if they can get by on one salary. There, unfortunately, lies the rub. The majority of dual-income couples working full time would gladly have one person change to part-time work or quit a job but feel that they can't manage without the extra income, or can they? The truth is that most couples can, depending on what hard financial choices they're willing to make.

To get an idea of whether you'll be able to get by on one income, do the following calculations:

Take what would be the sole earner's adjusted* monthly take-home pay:

$ _____,

Subtract your current total monthly household expenses:

- $ _____,

(Remove any monthly costs such as parking that are associated with the job you plan to eliminate.)

Total over/under your monthly income:

$ _____

A negative number indicates the amount of expenses you have to cut to break even living off one paycheck. A positive number means your family can survive on a single income, and you have the luxury of having one parent stay at home and provide full-time child care.

*Talk to your accountant to see if tax rates, insurance costs, and other payroll deductions can be modified to increase amount of your monthly take-home pay.

If being or having a SAHP is your goal, and you have to cut back on your expenses to live off one source of income, cutting out a latte here and there is not the best strategy; go after the bigger bucks. The items listed below signify large adjustments to a household's expenses. Don't get nervous while doing this exercise; you're not taking an oath of what you will do, but a look at what you could do. Once finished, look back at what you have left and ask yourself, would life be that bad with so much less?

Would you or your partner...	Yes!	Amount Saved
cancel part or all of your cable TV subscription?		
~~cancel your internet access~~?	no	
~~switch to a cheaper cell phone plan~~?	no	
stop or reduce contributions to a college or 401K fund?		
give up or greatly reduce meals out with friends?	yes	
cancel gym or club membership, plus any recreational classes?	yes	
give up all forms of gambling?		
drastically reduce use of air conditioner or heater?		
cancel or forgo any expensive vacations?		
cut your grocery bill in half?		
cut out the take-out and pack your lunch for work?		
carpool or take public transportation to work?		
do your own gardening, house cleaning, and pool cleaning?		

Would you or your partner...	Yes!	Amount Saved
sell a second car and get by with only one vehicle?		
trade in your car for a different model that's cheaper, and easier to maintain?		
modify or severely cut down the amount of insurance you carry?		
refinance a mortgage or other debts to make lower monthly payments?		
give up buying tickets to concerts or sporting events?		
cut any purchases related to a hobby (fishing, golf, crafting, etc.)?		
switch to a cheaper stylist and stop all beauty treatments (manicures, waxing, hair dyeing, tanning, etc.)?		
Total Saved	$	

Your total saved should be enough to eliminate any overspending of your monthly budget. With proper oversight of your expanses and a willingness to make some sacrifices, the luxury of choosing whether or not to be a SAHP could become an option.

How will you compensate your chosen care giver?

Even a SAHP needs a helping hand every now and then. How you plan to compensate a chosen care giver, even if it's only part-time, goes beyond the agreed-upon salary. When hiring a nanny or au pair (covered in Chapter 7), there are agency fees, payroll taxes, and stipend expenses in addition to the person's salary. If a friend or relative will be watching your child free of charge, consider at the very minimum the time and mileage spent dropping off and picking up your child from someone's home. The following questions will help you determine the true cost of using a care giver while clarifying what expenses you'll agree to cover.

1. If a friend or relative doesn't ask to be paid for watching your child, would you try offering some other form of compensation for his/her time and effort? If so, what would it be, and how hard would you try to make sure it was accepted?

2. If hiring a care giver from an agency, are you aware of all application and administrative fees due?

3. Will you provide insurance or any other benefits such as vacation pay?

4. Will you pay extra for working holidays or overtime?

5. What do you consider overtime?

6. Would you prefer to pay your care giver "under the table?"

7. Will you plan to give your care giver an end-of-year bonus?

8. How often, if at all, would you expect to give your care giver a raise?

9. Will you provide a stipend to cover incidental costs while caring for your child?

10. Will you deduct meal costs from your care giver's pay?

11. Will you reimburse your care giver for any entertainment costs, such as taking your child to the movies or to the zoo?

12. If your care giver accidentally breaks an appliance or valuable item, would you deduct the cost from her paycheck?

13. If your care giver mentions that the neighbor pays her more per hour, would you increase her pay to keep her, or stick with your agreed-upon lower rate?

14. Would you give your care giver an advance on her salary if she asked?

15. What would you do if you felt your care giver was not worth her salary but was the only person you could afford to hire?

With all the grumbling about the high cost of child care, it may come as a surprise to see the USDA's *Expenditures on Children by Families* (2011) report found that "Child care and education was the only budgetary component for which about half of all households reported no expenditure." The study goes on to explain that the higher a family's income, the more likely they are to spend money on child care, and the more they're willing to pay for this service. In reality, all parents pay for day care in one way or another; even those who get free day care from relatives or through a government program. There are transportation costs, birthday and holiday gift exchanges, or other incidentals frequently missed when calculating total care expenses.

How much will it cost to send your child to day care?

For parents that choose to enroll their child in a day care program, how much they pay varies greatly based on location. If you want to get an idea of what some parents shell out for daily daycare, the non-profit ChildCare Aware of America estimates annual fees paid for full-time care of an infant in a family child care home range from $4,000 to $12,350. Full-time care for a four-year-old is slightly less, falling within a range of $3,850 to $9,600. Of course, the only thing that matters is how much *you* can expect to pay if you decide to enroll your child in a day care facility. To find out, call or do a quick web search on a local center and inquire about fees listed below.

Day Care Cost Calculator	Cost $
Admission	_____
After hours care	_____
Registration fee	_____
Deposit	_____
Activity fee	_____
Late fee	_____
Fund raising budget	_____
Sick day allowance (covers alternative care when your child is sick)	_____
Misc. (transportation, supplies, incidentals)	_____
Average monthly expense	_____

There are also intangible costs to sending your child to day care. While some parents are wracked with guilt at the thought of leaving their child with relative strangers for hours, others find it a welcomed relief, and well worth the added expense. It's the emotional factors, those that pull at your heart strings—guilt, joy, freedom, tradition—that should also be considered along with those controlled by your purse strings.

What impact will your child's education have on your wallet?

Elementary through secondary public school systems in the U.S. spent an average of $10,615 per pupil in fiscal year 2010 (U.S. Census Bureau, 2012) to ensure your, and every other, child in America grows up knowing how to read, write, and do arithmetic. But your tax dollars will not cover all the expenses of a free public education. Parents are responsible for school supplies (including computers, if required), transportation, or uniforms required by the school. Private schools and home school programs receive no government assistance, so parents are responsible for all the costs involved with educating their child. Choosing the right school for your child is covered in more detail in Chapter 8, but you can get an idea how much dough you'll be rolling out by contacting a few primary schools in your area and finding out the answers to the questions below:

1. Does the school offer a detailed list of the expenses beyond tuition parents should be expected to pay per year?

2. Are there any hidden or "voluntary" fees throughout the year?

3. Are parents expected to pay for all field trip expenses?

4. How many books and school supplies are parents expected to purchase during the school year?

5. Does the school require parents to purchase uniforms?

6. Do parents have to pay a fee to enroll their child in an extracurricular activity or program?

7. How much time would you like to spend helping with class projects, field trips, or special events?

8. Are parents expected to contribute time or money during fund drives?

9. What are the school's refund policies if you decide to move your child to a different school?

10. Does the school offer financial aid, or are scholarships available through the school or other organizations?

11. Will you have the ability to get on a board or organization that can influence the school's financial decisions?

12. Is the school chronically under-funded or facing severe budget cuts that will force parents to pick up the slack?

Comparing the costs between different schools?

Parents who live in larger cities or suburbs often have the nerve-wracking chore of choosing between multiple schools in their area. If you'll be choosing between multiple programs, or simply deciding between sending your child to a public or private school, fill out the comparison table that follows. By laying out the cost differences between programs, you can better analyze how much of your family's budget you're willing (or able) to devote to your child's education.

School Cost Calculator

	School A	School B	School C
Annual Expenses			
Tuition			
Registration and application fees			
Health/safety fee			
Sports team expenses			
Extracurricular club expense			
Activity fee (field trip costs, equipment, lessons, etc.)			
Meals and snacks program			
Fund raising budget			
Sick day allowance (cost of staying home or hiring sitter when your child is sick)			
Multiple child or other discount			
Commuting costs (parking, bus fees, mileage)			
Uniform expense			
Other (tutors, additional courses, etc.)			
Total Annual Cost			

Will driving your child around drive you into debt?

"According to the most recent available federal data, women overall spend 64 minutes per day in a car. Single mothers spend 75 minutes a day in the car. And, married mothers with school-aged children spend 66 minutes a day driving — that is almost 17 solid days in the car. Mothers are now spending more time driving than the average parent spends on primary child care."

-NPTS and The Americans' Use of Time Project

Pick up, drop off, pick up, drop off, fill the tank, and repeat. The Surface Transportation Policy Project (STPP) determined that mothers make an average of five trips a day compared to the national average of four, and women (mostly moms) account for two-thirds of all trips to chauffeur people around—driving kids to soccer games or taking an older parent to the doctor. This may explain why there's enough food, magazines, water bottles, blankets, sports equipment, and kiddie crap in a family car to stock an around-the-world expedition. In the United States, mommy traffic accounts for 60 percent of all transportation, and commuting costs take up 14 percent of the average family's annual budget.

The chart that follows offers a hypothetical average day of driving around with your pre-schooler. With the help of a map site like Google Maps, calculate how many miles you'll be traversing during the day. If you feel you're racking up more miles than an Amtrak conductor, investigate ride-sharing programs, public transportation options, or limiting the amount of programs you'll sign your child up for.

How much will you be driving in a day?

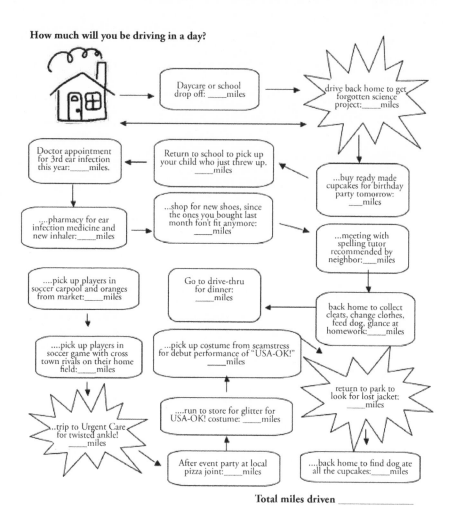

Daycare or school drop off: ____miles

drive back home to get forgotten science project:____miles

Doctor appointment for 3rd ear infection this year:____miles.

Return to school to pick up your child who just threw up. ____miles

...buy ready made cupcakes for birthday party tomorrow: ____miles

....pharmacy for ear infection medicine and new inhaler:____miles

...shop for new shoes, since the ones you bought last month don't fit anymore: ____miles

...meeting with spelling tutor recommended by neighbor:____miles

....pick up players in soccer carpool and oranges from market:____miles

Go to drive-thru for dinner: ____miles

back home to collect cleats, change clothes, feed dog, glance at homework:____miles

....pick up players in soccer game with cross town rivals on their home field:____miles

...pick up costume from seamstress for debut performance of "USA-OK!" ____miles

return to park to look for lost jacket: ____miles

..trip to Urgent Care for twisted ankle! ____miles

....run to store for glitter for USA-OK! costume: ____miles

After event party at local pizza joint:____miles

....back home to find dog ate all the cupcakes:____miles

Total miles driven _____

How much will it cost to feed your growing family?

"The average American family of four (married couple with two children) spent approximately $185 per week on food (away and at home) in 2009. This spending does not buy a nutritious diet…Contrary to popular opinion that a healthier diet costs more, it is possible for people to eat healthier, including more vegetables and fruits, and spend less on food."

-USDA, Eating Healthy on a Budget — The Consumer Economics Perspective, 2009

How much will you spend on groceries and eating out after you have your baby? Initially, not much, if you're counting on breast-feeding your infant. But what if this natural and free source of food doesn't pan out, or your child has dietary needs that require store-bought formula? Bottle-feeding your baby could add $80.00 a month to your grocery bill. Then, quicker than you can say "spit up," your baby will have graduated to solid foods, and then quickly morph into an around-the-clock eating machine. On average, a family will spend 16 percent of household expenses on food, most parents swearing that it all goes toward milk, Cheerios, and goldfish crackers.

Yet it's eating habits, not quantity eaten, that will determine how much you'll spend to feed your family. The USDA suggests following the three P's: plan, purchase, prepare (at home), to maintain a healthy diet on a modest income. This sounds like a good idea, but when you're trying to squeeze in lunches or dinners between swimming lessons, spelling drills, and laundry, you may resort to the three D's: done, delivered, or drive-thru.

To see if you're prone to practicing pricey feeding habits, answer the questions below:

1. Will you buy prepared baby food rather than make it yourself?

2. Would it be impossible for you to pass up a fro-yo shop, food court, or coffee kiosk without treating your child to a snack?

3. Will your favorite place to meet fellow mommies be at fast food restaurants with playgrounds?

4. Once your child can eat solids, will your chicken dinners usually come in a bucket, box, or served as nuggets?

5. Will you strictly buy organic produce at specialty shops?

6. Do you think coupons and reward programs are more of a bother than they're worth?

7. Could you see yourself ignoring any grocery lists or food budget you created to help save money?

8. Do you feel buying food staples in bulk and planning meals around supermarket sales are a waste of time?

9. When taking family trips to ball games, museums, or other outings, will you purchase meals and snacks at concession stands rather than packing food from home?

10. Will you be too embarrassed to apply for public assistance (WIC, EBT, free school meals), even if you qualify?

If the majority of your responses are "yes," you're literally spending more dollars for your doughnuts than necessary. By preparing and eating most of your meals and snacks at home, you'll not only train your child's taste buds to prefer foods without the added sugar, salt, and unpronounceable additives found in most pre-packaged and fast foods, but you'll also teach your child that *going out* doesn't automatically mean *eating out* somewhere.

How much baby stuff do you really need to buy?

"That idea that you can save money by using hand-me-downs was a myth! We have a box of cleats in the garage. Every time one of my kids needed cleats I'd say, 'Go to the box and grab a pair.' Of course, none of them ever fit right, or was the right type. So, off to the store we'd go to buy yet another pair of cleats that would get used for maybe one season and then thrown in the box with the rest."

-Scott, father of a 9-year-old daughter
and sons 12 and 16 years old

"There came a point where there were just too many toys. I admit I went a little overboard when one son showed an interest in a particular book, so I went out and bought the whole series. But the happiest day was when I gave them (the toys) all away. It was so liberating. Now that my boys are older, I see them learning while forming relationships. They didn't do this when they were younger, maybe because the toys were such a distraction."

-Tina, mother of four boys ages 4 to 14

There's no way around it, kids need stuff, and there's no shortage of books and websites offering long lists of "must have" baby items. If you're not careful, the amount you spend on baby stuff can get out of hand. A recent U.K. study discovered that expectant parents will spend close to £1,500 (around $2,400) on nursery products and essentials *before* their baby is born. Bump up that amount to approximately $7,000 spent by the baby's first birthday.

Admittedly, it's hard to resist the adorable outfits or feeling as if you're jeopardizing your child's mental and social development by not purchasing the right toys. An overwhelming number of new parents admit, in hindsight, to buying more baby goods than they needed or spending too much for what they did buy, despite their desire to be practical. Tempting as it is to add the entire catalog of Baby Einstein™ products into your shopping cart or to splurge on that $1,000 travel system, ask yourself the following question: Is this item necessary, and can it be borrowed or bought for less?

Can you successfully buy all the baby gear you need on a budget?

To see if you're susceptible to falling into the overspending trap, take the following quiz. Mark whether you believe the statements are myths or genuine money-saving ideas.

	True	False
1. It's best to stock up on baby clothes before your child is born because you won't have time to shop.		✓
2. Clothes from consignment shops are stained or worn out.		✓
3. A good pair of shoes is essential for proper infant foot growth.		✓
4. It's helpful to have at least one fancy baby outfit on hand for formal events.		✓
5. Avoid buying pull up bottoms until your baby starts crawling.		
6. It's best to buy outfits one size larger since your baby will be growing so fast.		✓
7. The cost of buying and washing cloth diapers cancels out any savings gained by using disposable diapers.		✓
8. You need intelligence-building toys to stimulate your baby's mind.		
9. Buying several different reading books will keep your child from becoming bored hearing the same story repeatedly.		✓
10. A crib mobile is necessary to build strong hand-eye coordination.		
11. Buying a "white noise" music player to help calm a fussy child is worth the cost.		✓
12. Avoid using second-hand car seats and cribs.	✓	
13. Any product described as an all-in-one solution will save you money because it's multipurpose.		
14. A baby wipe warmer, deodorant diaper disposal unit, and video monitor are essential for a well-stocked nursery.	✓	
15. It's best to wait until after your baby shower to purchase clothing for your baby.	✓	

Answers:

1. False. You won't know your child's size or how quickly he will grow to warrant stocking up on any particular size of clothing.

2. False. Many items are new with their original price tags attached.

3. False. Infants don't need shoes, so pass on this purchase.

4. False. Unless you plan to attend a wedding within the next few weeks, your baby may outgrow the outfit you've saved for a special occasion.

5. True. Onesies and drawstring gowns make for easier diaper changes. Once crawling, choose bottoms with snaps on the inseams and avoid dresses that get caught under the knees.

6. False. Buying the wrong size does not save you money and is uncomfortable and dangerous for your baby.

7. False, unless you use an expensive delivery service.

8. False. Pots, plastic bowls, and shoeboxes are just as stimulating to a toddler as a high-priced brain-building toy. Use the money you save to start a college savings plan.

9. False. It will only keep you from going crazy reading the same story. Children are content to hear you read their favorite book over and over again.

10. False. Your baby will have plenty of visual and muscle stimulation from other sources.

11. True, sometimes. While this tactic works on some babies, it has no effect on others—but you don't have to purchase a CD to find out if it's right for you. Record a running dishwasher or clothes dryer and play it back while your baby is fussy. If it works, you're set and you've saved some dough.

12. True. Although you could save money by using your cousin's old car seat, it may not be safe based on current standards. Unless it was originally purchased less than two years ago and is in pristine condition, buy new.

13. False. You could be paying for unnecessary features or find that it's cheaper to purchase individual items to do the same tasks. These types of items may also be too big and cumbersome or used for such a short period that it doesn't warrant the extra expense.

14. False. While these are all nice to have, they aren't essential. A good guide to follow before purchasing an item is to ask yourself, "Did my grandparents manage without this?" If they did, you can too.

15. True. The generosity of friends and relatives could keep you free from shopping for clothes and other essentials for months and may even save you the expense of big-ticket items. Whatever you didn't get at your shower, you could buy online and have delivered after your baby is born.

If you chose incorrectly more than twice, you may be choosing to be frivolous instead of frugal with your money.

What essential information should you know about your medical insurance coverage?

"Expected cost of maternity care without insurance: $2,000 prenatal care $6,000-$8,000 low-risk delivery in hospital; $10,000-$22,000 high-risk or cesarean delivery (American Pregnancy Association, 2011). Typical out-of-pocket costs for maternity care with insurance: under $500 - $3,000." (CostHelper.com, 2013)

With the passage of the Affordable Care Act, virtually all women and children will be covered by some form of medical insurance, whether purchased individually, provided by an employer, or granted by a government agency. How this will change the eight percent of a family's budget that goes toward medical expenses is for the future to reveal. Yet guaranteed coverage may not mean equal coverage from policy to policy, and few contracts cover 100 percent of all costs. Don't get caught owing whopping medical bills for services you thought were covered but were not. It's not only imperative that you know the details of your coverage—for example, whether all ultrasounds are covered, or 3-D imagery is excluded—but how much you can expect to pay in co-payments, parking, and other incidentals.

Review your current policy to see what percent of the following common maternity expenses are covered in the table that follows.

Insurance	100% Covered	Limited Coverage ($ or %)	Not Covered
Your Pregnancy			
Cost of commuting to appointment			
Prenatal vitamins			
Pregnancy books & videos			
Pregnancy yoga classes			
Anti-stretch mark creams			
Holistic anti-nausea treatments			
3-D images or video of ultrasound			
Prenatal acupuncture			
Your Delivery			
Doula			
Midwife			
Labor/birthing coach			
Private birth room in hospital			
Postpartum therapist			
Postpartum Care			
Circumcision			
Birthmark erasing			
Baby formula			
Light therapy			
Nursing bras, body wear			
Lactation specialist			
Pediatric Care			
Neonatal intensive care			
Autism treatment			
Physical therapy for your baby			
Chronic illness care (diabetes, asthma)			
Orthopedic products (leg, back braces)			

CHAPTER 3

Your Pregnancy

"When I was pregnant with my first daughter, my husband got morning sickness, but I was fine! He had headaches, nausea, and would vomit in the morning, which was so unusual. I just thought he was sick, and didn't make the association until I got pregnant for the second time and the same thing happened!"

-Rocio, mother of 35- and 36-year-old daughters and four adopted children ages 19-26 years old

Be happy humans aren't elephants. Our pregnancies usually last about 38 weeks after conception, while the pachyderms have to endure 22 months of crazy peanut cravings and feeling fat. Despite our comparatively short gestation, more books and articles are written about these precious nine months than the remaining 18 years of human parenting. The following section will explore the choices you can expect to make while you're expecting.

What type of maternity healthcare giver should you choose?

Obstetrician, doula, midwife or registered nurse? Stick with your current doctor, or find someone new? Having your first child is a big deal, involving lots of appointments and intimate exchanges. You certainly don't want to spend the next nine months with someone who isn't on your wavelength or whose opinions you don't trust. Recommendations from friends or a list of names provided by your insurance company may narrow the search, but whom should you choose? The following questions will help you decide what type of health care professional you want to become your confidant, instructor, and overseer during your amazing, life-giving transformation.

Should you stick with your family doctor or a general practitioner?

1. Do you prefer to work with a physician who has known and treated you for years?

2. Do you want a physician who can also serve as your child's general practitioner after birth?

3. Would you like to have a one-stop doctor that can manage your pregnancy, gynecological exams, and general care?

4. Are you confident that you will have a healthy pregnancy and delivery without complications?

Why choose an obstetrician/gynecologist?

1. Do you prefer to work directly with a physician who works in a hospital?

2. Will you likely have a high-risk pregnancy?

3. Does your insurance only cover maternity care provided by an OB/GYN?

4. Are you comfortable with the possibility of being tended to by an assistant during routine procedures or during labor?

If you answered "yes" to all the questions above, an OB/GYN may be the logical choice to provide care during your pregnancy and delivery. Unlike midwives and doulas, OB/GYNs can write prescriptions and perform c-sections and other advanced medical procedures.

Why choose a midwife?

1. Do you want to deliver your baby at home?

2. Are you likely to have a pregnancy with minimal medical intervention?

3. Do you prefer highly personal medical care?

4. Are you looking to increase your chances of having a vaginal birth?

If you answered "yes" to the questions above, perhaps you would like a midwife as your primary care giver or in addition to your physician. There are various types of midwives available. For example, a Certified Nurse Midwife (CNM) is a medical nurse with a college degree and training in midwifery, while a Certified Professional Midwife (CPM) may not have a degree, but has received extensive training in a professional midwife school. Some work alone, while others work along with physicians. Do your homework before arranging any interviews. Familiarize yourself with your state's regulations regarding this type of profession, and any restrictions your insurance policy may impose.

Why hire a doula?

1. Are you looking for someone to provide emotional support and educated guidance from the beginning of your pregnancy all the way through to the day you take your baby home?

2. Do you want to work with someone who specializes in a holistic approach to pain and stress management?

3. Is it important that you work with someone who will remain by your side even if you decide to change doctors or are referred to various specialists?

4. Are you looking for someone to provide practical and emotional guidance and support postpartum?

If you answered "yes" to the above questions, a doula will provide you with the extra care and attention you seek. Unlike OB/GYNs or CNMs, doulas cannot deliver your baby but will work with your physician and be a cherished advocate for your well-being.

What qualifications do you want in your care giver?

Love for a particular care giver is one thing; logistics is another. As wonderful as your feelings may be about a particular clinician, if commuting to her office is a hassle, or her office hours work against your schedule, you're more likely to cancel appointments or arrive stressed and flustered, neither of which are healthy during your pregnancy. This, along with the conditions in the questions below, should be considered when making your selection.

Considerations when choosing a maternity care giver:

1. Does she have experience with water births or alternative delivery methods that have been shown to be safe?

2. Is she licensed to perform home deliveries?

3. Is the care giver also a certified lactation consultant?

4. When do the care giver's services start and when do they end?

5. Does the care giver have permission to work at the facility where you plan on giving birth?

6. Will she do everything possible to ensure you have a vaginal birth?

7. Will she not be on vacation or maternity leave at any time during your pregnancy?

8. Is the care giver an active member of a professional organization like the American Board of Obstetrics and Gynecology (ABOG), Midwives Alliance of North America (MANA), or Doulas of North America (DONA)?

9. Has the care giver ever gotten in an argument with a hospital staff member or patient?

10. Does the care giver specialize in holistic treatments in addition to traditional medicine?

11. Who will be the backup care giver if she can't come to your assistance?

Considerations when choosing a pediatrician

While investigating and choosing maternity healthcare professionals, you will also need to select a pediatrician for your child, once born. Many hospitals require that you choose this physician before you deliver. As with your maternity care giver, choose carefully. You'll be going to quite a lot of appointments—possibly three or more in the first month after delivering—which makes ease of making appointments even more of a priority. Below are some points to ponder while deciding on the best pediatrician for your baby:

1. Is the physician so popular that scheduling an appointment is difficult?

2. How easy is it to book a next-day appointment?

3. Does the physician speak your native language well or with a heavy accent that makes her difficult to understand?

4. Has the physician ever been placed on medical probation or fined for medical misconduct?

5. Does the physician only work in your area a few days a week?

6. Would you prefer a physician that specializes in a genetic condition that could be passed on to your child?

7. How much time does the physician allot for each appointment?

8. Does the physician have a policy that cancels your appointment if you arrive late?

9. Will you be charged for a last minute appointment cancellation?

10. Will many duties be taken care of by an assistant or specialist and not the physician herself?

How closely will you watch what you eat while pregnant?

You want to eat healthy while pregnant, but with all the conflicting information being thrown around you're not sure what's safe. If sushi is a no-no while pregnant, what do pregnant Japanese women eat? In an effort to straighten out any confusion, a list of foods and beverages you may crave while pregnant are shown below. Enter the corresponding letter that indicates how safe you believe each item is to consume.

Is It Safe?

Y = Yes! Totally safe. M = OK in small amounts. N = Not safe at all.

hot dog	pepperoni pizza	veggie wrap with sprouts
_____	_____	_____
Ahi tuna salad	Caesar salad	salad with blue cheese dressing
_____	_____	_____
rare roast beef	beef jerky	beef bologna
_____	_____	_____
smoked salmon	raw oysters	grilled swordfish
_____	_____	_____
eggs over easy	Eggs Benedict	egg nog
_____	_____	_____
decaf coffee	cappuccino	mocha latte
_____	_____	_____

green tea _____	chai tea _____	raspberry tea _____
diet cola _____	diet shake _____	energy drink _____
one apple martini on a special occasion _____	one large beer a week _____	one shot of tequila a month _____
fresh pressed apple juice _____	organic raw milk _____	wheatgrass juice _____
homemade ice cream _____	cookie dough _____	unbaked mousse or meringues _____

Answers: According to the American Association of Pregnancy Health, none of the above are recommended for consumption because they contain at least one of the following: preservatives such as sodium nitrate (found in deli meats and smoked foods), raw or undercooked eggs, caffeine, alcohol, artificial sweeteners, or are foods with a high risk of carrying toxic bacteria that could cause illness and pregnancy complications. Review the list above with your healthcare professional who will be the ultimate word on what you can eat or drink and what you should avoid.

Will you be taking any drugs or supplements while pregnant?

For all the beauty and wonder that pregnancy promises to deliver, comfort is rarely mentioned in the same breath. Bloating, hemorrhoids, heartburn, varicose veins, nausea, and moodiness are only some of the annoying symptoms mommies-to-be may experience. Begging for relief, you may turn to a little chemical assistance to ease the pain. Will your pursuit of comfort come at the expense of your baby's safety?

Below are several remedies to common ailments. Enter the appropriate letter to indicate how safe you believe each option is to take while pregnant.

Is It Safe?
Y = Yes! Totally safe. M = OK in small amounts. N = Not safe at all.

Symptoms	**Remedies**		
Aches and pain	salicylate or acetylsalicylic acid (aspirin) ___	ibuprofen (Advil) ___	acetaminophen (Tylenol) ✓
Common cold	pseudoephedrine (found in Sudafed and other decongestants) ___	chlorpheniramine (found in Theraflu and other cold medicines) ___	menthol rub ___
Allergy relief	fluconazole (Sudafed) ___	nasal spray decongestants (Afrin, Nasonex) ✗	neti pot (saline nasal wash) ___
Nausea relief	Dimenhydrinate (Dramamine) ___	bismuth subsalicylate (Pepto-Bismol) ? ___	ginger ale ___
Heartburn	sodium bicarbonate (Alka Seltzer or products with baking soda) ___	aluminum hydroxide or aluminum carbonate (Maalox, Mylanta) ___	calcium carbonate (Tums) ___
Acne	tetracycline ___	salicylic acid ___	benzyl peroxide ___
Bloating & gas	natural charcoal pills ___	anti-gas tablets ___	peppermint leaves or tea ___
Constipation	laxative ___	enema ___	prunes & fiber pills ___
Depression	prescription antidepressants ___	herbal antidepressants ___	fish oil pills ___

surfak   metamucil   ___

magnesium citrate

63

Answers: In each symptom category, the first two remedies listed are not recommended during pregnancy, but the third option is completely safe. Again, your healthcare professional will be the ultimate judge as to what you can take for any ailments. If professional advice isn't available, and you're unsure whether you should pop a pill our drink a potion, follow this basic rule: When in doubt, don't.

Will you take risks to look ravishing?

Afraid to let people know you're not a natural blond? Does the fear of going au naturel have you considering completely secluding yourself for the next nine months? Which of the following beauty treatments are safe to indulge in while pregnant? Enter the letter in the table that follows that indicates how safe each treatment, product, or procedure is to use or have done while pregnant.

Is It Safe?

Y = Yes! Totally safe. M = OK in small amounts. N = Not safe at all.

perm _____	chemical straightener _____	blow out _____
gloss treatment _____	deep conditioner _____	hot oil treatment _____
all over color _____	highlights _____	henna rinse _____
tanning booth _____	self tanning lotion _____	bronzing makeup _____
laser hair removal _____	depilatory cream _____	shaving or waxing _____
full set acrylic nails _____	manicure pedicure _____	polish free buffing _____
enzyme body wrap _____	herbal oil massage _____	pregnancy massage _____
acupuncture _____	acupressure _____	foot rub _____

Answers: The items in the first two columns are considered unsafe to do while pregnant due to exposure to toxic chemicals or fumes. The third offers safer alternatives. Before doing any beauty treatment that involves a store-bought product, carefully read the label and talk to your clinician to verify its safety. If the label says it's not suitable for use while pregnant, set it aside. Let the flush of excitement and anticipation of giving birth be your beauty aid and skip the rest. A healthy baby will be your reward for tolerating months of frizzy hair with dark roots, and short nails.

Labor and leisure: What activities should you avoid while pregnant?

Just because you're pregnant, doesn't mean your home will clean itself or that you should lock yourself in your room and avoid all physical activity for the next nine months. Life goes on, and there are chores to do and fun to be had. Even if house cleaning has never been your top priority, you may be taken by the suddenly strong urge to redecorate, clean, and shop. Now that you have a baby on board, you should ask yourself if there are tasks that should be avoided. Should you remodel or simply redecorate to create a nursery? Should you join a walk-a-thon instead of a marathon? Take the quiz below by entering the letter that indicates how safe you think each activity is for pregnant women.

Is It Safe?

Y = Yes! Totally safe. M = OK in small amounts. N = Not safe at all.

using household
chemical cleansers _____

painting the
nursery _____

making tie-dye
crafts _____

changing the cat's
litter box _____

using insect
repellants
or pesticide
sprays _____

repotting or
fertilizing
plants _____

swimming in a
ocean, lake, or river _____

soaking in a
hot tub _____

taking a long
bubble bath _____

jogging _____

horseback
riding _____

off-road
driving or
biking _____

flipping your
mattress _____

carrying heavy
groceries _____

moving
furniture _____

Answers: None of the activities listed above are recommended for a pregnant woman. The first two rows should be avoided due to exposure to toxic fumes or microorganisms that can find their way into a pregnant woman's system and cause complications. Likewise, microbes or chemicals (perfumed soaps, pollution) found in bodies of water may pose a risk to your pregnancy, as can high water temperatures, which means trips to the sauna and electric blankets are all no-nos. As for the physical activities listed on the last two rows, any endeavor that requires heavy lifting or subjects the body to constant pounding or joggling puts too much stress on your uterus and surrounding muscles and could bring on premature labor.

Inform your clinician if you feel you can't avoid any of the activities listed above. If you're certain you can't turn over chores that involve strong chemicals or active organic compounds (always read labels) to someone else, take all the necessary precautions—wearing gloves, facemask, and washing your hands and clothing thoroughly afterwards. Risky recreational activities should be easier to curtail. An hour-long nap will be more appealing than an hour-long jog when you're seven months pregnant and feeling huge. As for your beloved evening bubble bath, keep the water warm, not hot, and skip the suds.

Could you have a high-risk pregnancy?

"I had A LOT of pregnancy complications. I had gestational diabetes and high blood pressure, even though I was healthy. I followed doctor's orders even when he said a glass of wine would help take the stress off the baby by allowing me to relax. I was on bed rest for four months and only allowed one piece of fruit a day; I had a hard time sticking to one piece...What helped most during my pregnancy was the pool. My high-risk doctor suggested it to take the pressure off."

-Heather, mother of a 7-year-old son

Overall, 90-95 percent of all pregnancies progress normally and in good health, but recently the number of high-risk pregnancies has started to climb. Partly responsible for this increase is our modern lifestyle—consuming more calories than we can burn off, and modern medicine—enabling women who otherwise would be unable to conceive or carry a fetus full-term to bear a child with the help of pharmaceuticals. Fortunately, the majority of all high-risk pregnancies end with successful deliveries of healthy babies, thanks to early recognition of the risk factors and proper treatment. If you're unsure if you're a candidate for a high-risk pregnancy, answer the questions below:

Are you overweight?

1. Is your calculated BMI (Body Mass Index*) over 25?
2. Have you been overweight for most your life, or did you gain most your weight within the last few years?

3. Is there a family history of obesity, or are other members of your immediate family overweight?

4. Will you be trying to lose weight while pregnant?

5. Have you had gastric bypass surgery, or are you currently on an herbal supplement program to help you lose weight?

6. In addition to being overweight, do you suffer from diabetes, high blood pressure (hypertension), or other conditions related to being overweight?

7. Even if you don't have the conditions mentioned above, do members of your immediate family suffer from any of those conditions?

If you answered "yes" to any of the questions above, you may have increased risk for gestational diabetes (and its complications such as preeclampsia), gestational hypertension, extreme morning sickness, and other complications. Your OB/GYN will devise a program for you to follow to ensure you have the safest pregnancy possible.

*Ask your physician or go to *http://www.cdc.gov/healthyweight/assessing/bmi/* to calculate your BMI.

Are you a smoker?

1. Have you concluded that you're unable to quit smoking while pregnant?

2. Do you believe the best you can do is cut back on the number of cigarettes you smoke daily while pregnant?

3. Do you believe that the stress of quitting cold turkey will be worse than continuing to smoke?

4. Do you plan to use nicotine patches or gum during your pregnancy to help you cut back or quit smoking?

5. Even if you quit, will you be around other smokers or regularly exposed to second-hand smoke?

6. Will you be exposed to third-hand smoke (the smell and ashes that linger in a smoker's car, room, or clothing)?

If you answered "yes" to any of the above, you're at a higher risk for having placenta placement problems, gestational hypertension, or slow-developing fetus. If quitting or keeping away from smokers is not an option, it's important that you choose a health practitioner who is easy to visit and readily available, since you'll need to be monitored closely during your pregnancy.

Are you more than 35 years old?

1. Did you recover from a serious accident that occurred when you were younger?

2. Do your job or other obligations or situations make your life very stressful?

3. Has it been more than five years since your last physical or gynecological exam?

4. Have you had one or more serious illnesses in your lifetime?

If you answered "yes" to any of the questions above, these factors combined with your age may put you at a higher risk for complications such as early labor, placental problems, and even miscarriage.

Do you have hypertension or diabetes, or have a family history of these diseases?

1. Will you be taking medication to monitor these conditions while pregnant?

2. Have your lifestyle choices contributed to your having any of these diseases?

3. Did your own mother or any sisters have pregnancy complications due to having these conditions?

4. Despite having a family history with these diseases, have you been able to avoid coming down with any of these illnesses?

If you answered "yes" to any of the above questions you're at a higher risk for developing gestational diabetes and hypertension, or having a fetus that grows too large for a vaginal delivery. In addition to monitoring your fetus's healthy development, your doctor will ensure any treatment does not put your health at risk during gestation.

Do you have a higher-than-average chance of catching a viral or bacterial infection?

1. Have you NOT been inoculated against measles, mumps, and chicken pox?

2. Do you avoid getting an annual flu shot?

3. Do you work in a day care, a hospital, or medical clinic?

4. Are you an avid gardener, farmer, or do you live with multiple cats or other animals?

5. Have you had multiple sexual partners?

If you answered "yes" to any of the above questions, you may be exposing yourself to highly contagious infectious diseases that can affect your fetus's growth or cause premature labor. If you're not already pregnant, speak with your doctor about getting the shots you need or to treat any infections you may currently have. While pregnant, limit your exposure to the elements mentioned above while following strict personal hygiene habits.

Are you underweight, do you have a poor diet, or are you recovering from a recent serious illness?

1. Do you frequently feel weak or tired, yet have difficulty getting a good night's sleep?

2. Are your gums more white than pink, or have you ever been diagnosed as anemic?

3. Are you taking post-surgery medications, or prescription drugs for a chronic condition?

4. Are you recovering from the effects of chemotherapy or transplant surgery?

5. Are you anorexic, bulimic, or following a radical diet to lose weight?

If you answered "yes" to any of the above questions your fetus may be at risk for slow or improper growth in your womb, or to be born prematurely. A poor diet can also compromise your immune system, making you and your fetus susceptible to dangerous infections. Ask your OB/GYN if she feels a referral to a nutritionist would be beneficial.

Have you had recent gynecological surgery or an abortion before your pregnancy?

1. Have you ever had a LEEP procedure to treat a problem with your cervix?

2. Have you ever been treated for an ectopic pregnancy?

3. Have you recently had a surgical abortion?

If you answered "yes" to any of the questions above, there may be pregnancy risks associated to the treatment you received. It's best that your OB/GYN have as much information as possible about your treatment, including contact information for those who provided care, so proper decisions are made about how to manage your pregnancy.

What if you found out you were pregnant with multiples?

Automatically considered a "high risk" pregnancy, finding out you'll be carrying not one, but two (or more!) lovely little souls inside your womb is both thrilling and frightening. To help dispel any myths and bring you to a better understanding on how a pregnancy with multiples is different from one with a singleton, take the little quiz below.

Which of the following statements about being pregnant with multiples are True and which are False?

	True	False
Most pregnancies of multiples don't run the full 40 weeks.	___	___
Women who are pregnant with multiples need to gain more weight faster than women pregnant with a singleton.	___	___
The range of weight to reduce the number of complications is smaller than that of a singleton pregnancy.	___	___
The amount of weight you gain in the first 28 weeks of your pregnancy is the most important.	___	___
It's easier to gain weight earlier in the pregnancy than later when the babies are larger and tend to push up against the stomach.	___	___
Your doctor may suggest eating every three to four hours if pregnant with twins and every two hours if carrying triplets or more, whether you're hungry or not.	___	___
When pregnant with multiples, it's OK to indulge in high-fat foods such as milk shakes, grilled cheese sandwiches, and frozen yogurt.	___	___
Not drinking enough water during a multiples pregnancy can lead to an early delivery.	___	___
Women pregnant with multiples are two to three times more likely to develop gestational diabetes than women pregnant with singletons.	___	___
Women pregnant with multiples may need more folic acid than what is provided in an over-the-counter prenatal vitamin.	___	___

Answers: All of the above are true. Mothers blessed with multiples are also blessed with being able to eat more and gain more weight. On the less indulgent side, they frequently suffer worse morning sickness and must visit their doctors more often. Many OB/GYNs refer patients expecting multiples to high-risk pregnancy specialists who have more experience with the medical conditions and nuances involved.

Pregnancy Survival Kit Checklist

☐ Pregnancy/birth ball

☐ Anti-nausea snacks, tea, or wristband

☐ Body pillow

☐ Belly- and back-supporting underwear

☐ Stretch mark cream

☐ Maternity jeans or leggings

☐ Comfortable slip-on flat shoes

☐ Video, book, or app with pregnancy-safe yoga poses

CHAPTER 4

Your Delivery

What should you expect during your delivery?

"With my first delivery, my doctor scheduled me to get induced since I was showing signs of preeclampsia during a normal weekly appointment. Since it was my first child, I had no idea what to expect. I was really hoping to be woken up by labor but that didn't happen. My labor was about 16 hours. My daughter was three weeks early and came out four pounds eight ounces. She was healthy, no complications at all. My second child was an easy birth. I got to experience labor pains and I had her within three hours. She was six pounds and seven ounces—so different from my first!"

-Coleen, mother of 3- and 8-year-old daughters

With all the labor horror stories thrown around by expectant mothers it's no wonder some women become terrified about crossing the finish line. This fear is so common; it warrants its own name: *tokophobia*.

Not only is unbearable pain a top concern, but leaving a doo-doo on the delivery table or being an uncontrollable screamer also rank high on the list. Apparently, it's easier to get over an episiotomy than an embarrassment. Educating yourself about the details of labor and delivery is one way to stop shaking in your boots about putting your feet in the stirrups. Choose the best answer to the questions below, and see how high you score in your knowledge of basic delivery facts.

Labor Quiz

1. What are the three stages of labor?

   a) Dilation of cervix, birth of infant, passage of placenta.

   b) Cramping, pushing, and screaming.

2. How long does Stage 1 last?

   a) Anywhere from a few hours to a few days.

   b) It's over within seconds.

3. How long does Stage 2 last?

   a) Up to eight hours.

   b) Up to eight minutes.

4. How long does Stage 3 last?

   a) A few minutes to a few hours.

   b) You should be done by your second push.

5. What are some techniques that help ease labor pains?

   a) Sitting in warm water, lying on your side, breathing exercises, listening to soothing music.

   b) Nothing you try will help the unbearable pain you'll feel.

6. What is the "Transition" labor phase, and why is it considered the most difficult time during labor?

    a) It's the time between Stage 1 and 2 when contractions are the strongest and women often feel irritable, nauseous, and at their wits' end.

    b) It's the time right after delivery when women feel the most fatigue.

7. How long after you begin feeling contractions should you check into your birthing center?

    a) When the contractions are close to five minutes apart and last around 30 seconds long.

    b) Immediately after feeling the first contraction.

8. Will your water break before or after your labor contractions begin?

    a) Your amniotic sac could tear before, during, or after contractions begin, or not until ruptured by your physician.

    b) Your amniotic sac will always break right before contractions begin.

9. What are Braxton Hicks contractions?

    a) False labor contractions that help the body prepare for actual labor and delivery later on.

    b) Contractions that last longer than average.

10. What is a Bishop Score, and what does it help determine?

    a) A five-point vaginal examination to determine if labor will need to be induced.

    b) An examination of a mother's body temperature to determine the risk of overheating during labor.

11. What's a mucus plug?

    a) A mucus formation at the entrance of your cervix that can pop out hours, days, or weeks before labor.

    b) The heavy production of mucus that plugs a women's nose during labor, making it difficult to breathe.

12. How long after your due date could you be allowed to wait before labor is induced?

    a) Up to two weeks.

    b) Just one or two days.

13. What is a breech position?

    a) When the baby is in a butt- or feet-first position before labor.

    b) When a baby is in a horizontal position in the womb.

14. What can you do to lower your chance of having an unwanted cesarean (c-section) delivery?

    a) Choose a healthcare provider and facility that has a low cesarean rate and take childbirth classes.

    b) Bury a whole clove of garlic under a pine tree during a full moon.

The correct answer to all the questions is option "a." If you chose option "b" for most questions, you'll need more than this book to get your facts straight. When doing research, only visit sites from trusted sources such as the American Pregnancy Association's site, www.americanpregnancy.org, or the U.S. Department of Health and Human Services' site, www.womenshealth.gov. Misinformation is rampant on the Internet and could fuel your fears and misconceptions about labor and delivery. Your clinician or a trusted medical professional can also provide you with a list of websites, videos, and other sources of information that are trustworthy and accurate.

Where should you have your baby?

Not all babies are born in hospitals, nor, as Hollywood would like you to believe, in the back of taxicabs, or on a desk in a fancy office. Although the majority of babies are born in hospitals, every year thousands of women choose to give birth at home or in birthing centers. If you're able to choose where you will give birth (as opposed to being told where by your insurance company), factors such as cost, convenience, comfort, as well as any special services should all be considered. The detailed questions below may shed light on options that may influence your ultimate decision.

1. Does the facility have a higher-than-average rate for deliveries that develop complications?

2. Does the facility offer basic (level 1), intermediate (level 2), or advanced (level 3) neonatal care?

3. Will you be transferred to another hospital if you develop complications during delivery, or if your baby needs intensive care?

4. How many nurses or assistants are assigned to an expectant mother during labor and delivery?

5. Will you be transferred to different rooms during the different stages of labor?

6. Will you be sharing a delivery room? If so, with how many other patients?

7. Are family members allowed to assist or witness the birth of your baby?

8. Does the facility allow video recordings to be made of the delivery?

9. Does the facility offer different delivery methods, such as water births, (delivering while in a tub of warm water) or Leboyer-style births (delivering in a quiet, darkened room)?

10. Will the facility be doing major renovations around the time of your due date that could make rooms scarce or limit access to a snack shop, other amenities?

11. If you're traveling, do you know the location of nearby hospitals with an obstetrical department? (Not all hospitals have this department.)

12. On average, are women discharged and sent home soon after delivery?

13. What are the hospital's visiting hours and policies regarding the number of visitors and acceptable gifts or food that can be brought to the building?

14. Does the facility have personnel specifically trained or experienced in delivering multiples?

15. If you're opting for a home delivery, is your house conducive to a safe delivery and close to a hospital in the event there are complications during your delivery?

Will you have a friend or relative help you during labor and delivery?

You and your partner are one heck of a team, and together you can move mountains, but will he be your rock during delivery? It's nice wanting to share the miracle of childbirth with loved ones, but will a crowded delivery room hamper medical staff? Could your best friend be a fiasco in the delivery room?

Stories of birth partners fainting, tripping nurses, or becoming belligerent are all too common.

Safety, not sharing, should be the priority when deciding who will be in the delivery room at the time you're giving birth. The following questions should be considered before asking anyone to be your birth buddy. Once you've found someone who's up to snuff, your answers will help explain your expectations, should they agree to take on the job.

1. Is it important that your birth partner be a blood relative instead of a close friend?

2. Has someone shown a keen interest in being your birthing partner, or are you thinking of asking someone who has never mentioned the subject?

3. Do you want a birth partner to accompany you to your prenatal checkups or Lamaze classes?

4. Will you have a backup in case your chosen partner can't be with you when you go into labor? Will this backup receive the same training as your primary birth partner?

5. Will you allow your birth partner to help you deliver if she had a contagious illness such as a cold?

6. Can you count on your chosen birth partner to be available at a moment's notice, even if you go into labor in the middle of the night or far from home?

7. What will you do if your partner passes out at the sight of you giving birth?

8. Will you prefer *not* to have a birth partner, and to only be attended by professional healthcare workers?

9. Do you want a group of people to be your support team during labor and the delivery instead of one person?

10. How will you make sure that there won't be a clash of helpers, all trying to take charge during your delivery?

While some women want to share the experience of childbirth, bodily fluids and all, with loved ones, others find the thought of panting, pushing, and screaming, stark naked, in front of an audience horrifying. Choosing a birth partner is, like many other choices during pregnancy, highly personal. Select a person who wants to be there as much as you want that person by your side. If you feel the graphic nature of delivery is too much for some to witness, limit their assistance to the first stages of labor. The birth of your firstborn is not a time to shy away from being selfish. Do what's best for you, even if it may mean hurting someone's feelings.

What are your medical delivery options?

After a hormonal binge on pickles and ice cream, you have a crazy dream. You're in the hospital. Contractions are minutes apart and getting stronger. It's D-day. A nurse comes into your room with a contraption you've only seen in sci-fi movies. Moments later, yet another high-tech device appears, which, like the other, is supposed to monitor you and the baby. A second nurse hands you a menu with epidural, oxytocin, and episiotomy written in script under the heading "appetizers." You wake up, your head spinning. Will you be surrounded by NASA-worthy gadgets and forced to make medical decisions while in labor when all you can think about is whether or not it's OK to push?

"There's no such thing as a totally natural birth. If you're going to deliver in a hospital, there will always be some level of technology used during your labor and delivery, but that's a good thing," states Ana Lopes, M.D. and mother of two. "It's for your and your baby's safety."

Whether you want to give birth with aids only slight more advanced than a shoe string, some towels, and boiling water, or will only feel safe with a room full of high-tech machines, familiarize yourself with the various tests, treatments, and technology that will be available to you. What follows are several commonly used to deliver a baby. Discuss their benefits, risks, and necessity with your clinician to educate yourself about when and why, and if the procedures will be used during your intrapartum care.

Will the following be used during and after your labor and delivery? Y = Yes, it's a routine procedure O = Only if required or requested	Y	O
Fetal and uterine monitoring		
External fetal Doppler. A handheld ultrasound machine used to measure fetal heartbeats		
Tocometer. An instrument used externally to measure uterine contractions		
Biophysical profile (BPP). Ultrasound procedure that evaluates fetal breathing, movement, reflex, and amniotic fluid levels		
Intrauterine pressure catheter (IUPC). A small, flexible tube placed inside the uterus to measure contractions		
Fetal scalp electrodes (FSE). Small electrodes placed directly on the baby's head to monitor heart beats during labor		
Pain Management		
Epidural		
Spinal block		
Sterile papules (injections of warm water under the skin of the lower back to manage pain)		
Medication (Demerol, morphine, Stadol) delivered through IV or by shot		
Acupuncture/acupressure		

Labor Induction		
AROM (Artificial Rupture of Membrane). Physician tears amniotic sac or "breaks the water" to induce labor or aid delivery		
Membrane sweep. Physician sweeps your cervix with a finger to separate membranes and induce labor		
Chemical labor induction (drugs such as oxytocin, prostaglandin) administered through IV, shot, or direct placement on cervix)		
Vaginal Delivery Assistance		
Episiotomy. A surgical cut made to enlarge your vaginal opening		
IV medication (pain management, sedation, or medicinal)		
IV hydration (no drugs)		
Vaginal stretching massage		
Breech Plan		
Vaginal delivery preferred		
Cesarean delivery preferred		
Postpartum Requests		
Banking of umbilical cord blood		
Saving the placenta (if allowed)		
Eye drops and vaccination		
Circumcision (if baby is male)		

Should you create a cesarean plan?

In one word, "yes." Much has been written about the increasing frequency of cesarean births or c-sections. Close to one-third of all babies are born using this procedure. Which is why you should be prepared. The uptick in surgical deliveries can be attributed to the higher number of women delivering multiples, being over 35-years-old, or having health concerns during their pregnancy. While it has been suggested that doctors and expectant mothers opt for c-section out of convenience, most physicians and hospitals will only perform them if medically necessary.

Regardless of whether you decide to have a c-section ahead of time or find yourself unexpectedly being prepped for the procedure during labor due to complications, it's best to know the facts about cesareans before your delivery date.

Are the following facts about cesarean procedures true or false?

	T	F
The most common reasons for having a planned cesarean are the health condition of mother, a very large fetus, or the delivery of multiples.	_____	_____
The most common reasons for an emergency cesarean are: fetal distress during labor, placenta detachment before labor, dangerous position of fetus or umbilical cord.	_____	_____
Regarding a cesarean surgery, closing the incisions takes up more time than delivering the baby.	_____	_____
There are different types of incision that can be used for a cesarean delivery, each with its own advantages and disadvantages.	_____	_____

	T	F

Having a cesarean exposes a woman to the same risks of infection, blood clots, and damaged organs as found with other types of abdominal surgery.

_____ _____

Once a woman has a cesarean, she may be able to deliver future children vaginally.

_____ _____

To prepare a patient for a cesarean, an IV is inserted to administer a sedative, and a catheter is inserted to allow the patient to urinate during and after the surgery.

_____ _____

Women having a cesarean can choose to stay awake (not be anesthetized) and watch the procedure.

_____ _____

The normal recovery time for a cesarean is several days longer than that of a vaginal delivery.

_____ _____

The chemical and physical benefits unique to passing through the birth canal are not received if the baby is delivered by cesarean.

_____ _____

All of the facts above are true. Common as c-sections may become, they are still surgery and possess the same risks as any procedure that requires going under the knife. Discuss the details of this form of delivery and all your available options with your clinician. Be clear about how much risk you're willing to take on whether you're choosing a cesarean by choice or trying to avoid one in favor of a vaginal delivery.

What should you do if your baby has to stay in the hospital?

"Due to a medical emergency, my baby was delivered at 22 weeks. I was told she had a 10 percent chance of survival. I called my pastor to baptize my child. Through it all I was very calm. I thought, come what may, I want the knowledge that I did everything possible for my daughter. I know I couldn't achieve that feeling if I was not in a rational state of mind. I did not want to regret doing this or asking about that because I was overcome by the situation.

At home I was feeling full of despair after learning there was nothing else the doctors could do to save my daughter's life. I spoke to a family member and told her the news. She said 'Leave your emotions at the door before you enter the hospital. You can't let her feel your sadness, only your strength.'

When my baby was delivered, her fingers were webbed and her eyes were closed. It was amazing to watch her develop outside the womb. She was born December 21st. Four surgeries and over four months later, we left the hospital on April 21st. Today she's a normal, healthy eight-and-a-half-year-old."

-Lenice, mother of an 8-year-old daughter

Infants can sense your emotions while in the NICU, so your attitude is critical to your baby's recovery. In the opinion of Casey M. Calkins MD, author of *Fetal Surgery: Maternal-Fetal Intervention*, counseling the parents is almost as important as the procedures themselves. It is during these times of crisis that a child needs a parent who can stand up with confidence and can offer positive, loving support despite feeling like their world is ending in a tsunami of tears.

Successfully coping with the unfamiliar and hectic surroundings of a hospital's NICU department begins with gathering important information. As you approach your due date, tour your possible NICU department to familiarize yourself with the machines and staff members that work in the area, Further expand your knowledge by asking a supervisor the following questions:

1. What are the facility's visiting hours for parents and guests?
2. How often will you be given updates on your baby's condition?
3. If commuting back and forth from the hospital is difficult, will you be able to find lodging nearby?
4. Is there a Ronald McDonald house or other charitable lodgings that offer support for parents with a child in the NICU?
5. Does a separate team of doctors and staff work with babies in the NICU, or will your own doctor be providing care?
6. Does the department have on-site or on-call support counselors for parents?
7. Who will be your main contact if you have questions about your baby's condition?
8. Does the hospital provide literature about your baby's condition or a guide to all the machinery in the NICU ward?
9. Does the NICU encourage parents to hold their baby close to their bodies, as with kangaroo care?
10. If you don't like a particular staff member, will the facility quickly find a replacement?

Finding out your child has to spend one or more nights in the hospital is hard to hear, but not necessarily bad news. About 15 percent of all babies born spend time in a hospital's Neonatal Intensive Care Unit (NICU), most due to low birth weight as opposed to having an incurable or life- threatening disease, and 30-35 percent stay for under four days.

What if the absolute worst should happen?

Nobody wants to think of, let alone prepare for, the absolute worst way a pregnancy could end. No amount of preparation nor words of consolation will help a parent whose baby is stillborn or dies shortly after delivery. It's unlikely that you'll have to deal with such tragedy, but if fate were to force your hand, ask yourself if you would like any of the requests suggested below to be granted. Having a prepared list of requests available to give to hospital staff will make you better equipped to have your wishes executed at a time when it will be hard to think straight.

Bereavement Instructions

In the event of a loss _____ and _____ would like the following requests granted:

☐ To hold the baby for as long as possible (inquire ahead of time how long this will be).

☐ A private room to spend time with our deceased child and to mourn.

☐ Family members to be allowed to see our baby.

☐ To have the following name, _____, included in any relevant hospital documents.

☐ To keep the following mementos:

   ____lock of our baby's hair, _____medical bracelet, _____picture, _____ blanket or ID bracelet used at the hospital, _____ ink foot or hand prints

☐ Our child to be baptized immediately (provide contact name and info of preferred cleric performing ceremony).

☐ A blood sample drawn for genetic or zygosity testing.

☐ An autopsy or NO autopsy performed.

☐ To have our baby's body for private funeral arrangements.

☐ To donate our baby's body for scientific research.

☐ That anesthesia NOT be given during the delivery.

Delivery Day Checklist

- ☐ **Change of clothes.** You'll get sweaty and messy during labor and may have to stay overnight after delivery.
- ☐ **Slippers or slipper socks.** Got to keep your tootsies warm while your feet are in stirrups.
- ☐ **Small towel or wash cloth.** Sweaty and messy, remember?
- ☐ **Robe or cropped cotton cardigan.** Not too long or bulky.
- ☐ **Snacks**. You need fuel to keep up your energy.
- ☐ **Mouthwash or breath mints**. After panting for hours these will be godsend items.
- ☐ **Toiletry bag.** Include toothbrush, deodorant, makeup, hair bands, contact solution. (You'll want to freshen up and spruce up for all those pictures).
- ☐ **Sanitary napkins**. The fluids don't stop after the delivery.
- ☐ **Music playlist.** Listening to soothing music will calm your nerves and distract you during painful contractions.
- ☐ **Designated baby- or pet-sitter.** For those family members that can't be left alone.
- ☐ **Birthing Ball**. Looks like an exercise ball and helps position your body to control the pain.
- ☐ **Photographer/videographer.** Give one person this task and tell the others to put their cameras aside until after you delivered.
- ☐ **Your birth plan.** The list of procedures you want done or withheld if the need arises.
- ☐ **Proof of insurance,** ID or any other pertinent documents. There are always forms to fill out asking for this information.
- ☐ **Regulation-passing car seat.** Some hospitals won't release you without proof of ownership.

CHAPTER 5

Delivery of a Different Kind

"Mommies can have babies either from their tummies or from their hearts...So she had me from her heart."

–Jackie Danforth, adopted daughter of
TV journalist/producer Barbara Walters

Bringing home a baby delivered through the adoption process or with the help of a donor through Assisted Reproductive Technology (ART) has enabled millions of couples to establish beautiful families of their own. The world of adoption has truly gone global and traversed social boundaries as well. There's no doubt that starting a family through these channels brings on an additional set of unique questions. Despite your thorough research of agencies and clinics (and being thoroughly researched yourself), here are some questions or thoughts you may have missed during the process:

Have you covered the following details with your adoption or ART agency?

1. Are any of the final adoption or conception contracts or details handled by a "sister" agency?

2. If adopting, whose names are already on your baby's birth certificate (if one exists)?

3. Can your agency provide documentation on how thoroughly they checked the validity of your donor's claims or a referral's medical history?

4. Will you be informed about any existing or future offspring produced by your chosen donor?

5. Will you be notified if your donor later develops or discovers that he/she is a carrier of a genetic disease?

6. How much post-birth/adoption support does your agency provide?

7. Will there be any additional fees or expenses that pop up as you get closer to the delivery or relinquishment date?

8. Has the agency explained your rights as an expectant parent and the revocation laws in your state?

9. If the adoption does not go through, are the fees refunded or rolled over to the next attempted placement?

10. What's the refund policy if you decide to terminate your contract with your current agency or switch to another?

What are some considerations before accepting an adoption referral?

Receiving an adoption referral is both exciting, nerve-racking, and heartbreaking if you feel you wouldn't be the best parent for the child presented. A good agency will never force you to take a referral or look down on you if you pass on one. The questions below highlight considerations when going through this highly emotional phase of the adoption process.

1. What steps will you take to keep a level head during the very emotional event of meeting, accepting, or declining a referral?

2. If you've flown to a foreign country to meet a referral, would you feel pressured to accept the child because you couldn't afford the time or money to make another trip?

3. Can you employ an independent adoption physician to examine your child before accepting the referral?

4. If your child were ill at the time of your meeting, would you gladly take on the costs and management of treating the illness?

5. Are there any conditions or scenarios that, difficult as it may be, would have you decline a referral?

6. If you decline a referral, how long will it be until you are shown another?

7. Has there been a serious illness in this child's past? If so, how will this affect the child's current or future health?

8. What are the chances an aunt, grandparent, or other relative will challenge the adoption of this particular child?

9. How will you respond to a referral that had very limited medical information and little was known about his/her biological families?

10. Will you be allowed to spend more time with a referral if you felt it was needed before you could make a decision?

How can you make your foreign-born, adopted child feel comfortable in her new home?

Although they may only be days or months old, infants retain a memory of the sounds and scents of their birth country. The rhythm and inflections of the native language, the composition of the local diet, are different than what they will experience with their new, forever families. Below are questions aimed at easing the transition of bringing home a baby born in a foreign land.

1. Can you find out if your child has any allergies or aversions to certain foods?

2. Did your child have a favorite type of food, toy, or game that you could replicate at home?

3. Does the child have any strong fears of people, places, or things?

4. If your child had little interaction with other children or people, will you limit the number of visitors coming through your house?

5. If your child usually spent his/her time in a room full of other children, and your baby finds this comforting, how will you try to replicate that environment?

6. Will you learn to speak your child's native language or hire care-giving help that can speak your child's native language?

7. Will you load up on foods, books, clothes, and toys from your child's birth country?

8. Will you teach your child about his/her birth culture throughout his/her life, or only if he/she shows an interest?

9. Will you go out of your way to make friends with parents who are from or have children of the same culture as your child?

10. Will you always describe your child's birth country in positive terms?

Expectations should be thrown out when bringing home your adopted child. The milestones and developmental target dates set for babies born domestically should not be applied to those foreign born. To help their child flourish, parents should focus on providing love and comfort to their baby who not only has to adjust to new parents, but a new country as well.

What type of relationship are you expecting to have with the birth or donor parent?

> *"I get it. He's their biological father and all that crap. I mean, aren't we enough?"*
>
> -Nicole Allgood, mother of two donor children in the movie, *The Kids Are All Right*

In the movie quoted above, the parents of children conceived with donated sperm grapple with the unfamiliar task of forming a relationship with the newly discovered donor. Should they become friends with this biological connection to their children, and how much contact is healthy for their family? If you will be engaging in an open adoption or have contact with your child's biological donor, these types of questions, along with those below, should be considered.

1. How much contact would you like to have with your child's birth/ donor parent(s)?
2. Will you be withholding identifying information about a biological parent until your child reaches a certain age?

3. Will you try to alter your child's birth certificate to hide information about a biological parent?

4. What if you expected minimal contact with the donor/birth parent, but your child kept pressing for a closer relationship with his biological parent?

5. What if the donor/birth parent started becoming more involved in your child's life than you planned?

6. What if you have a falling out with the donor/birth parent later in life, and how will this affect your child?

7. If you agreed to have regular contact with your child's birth parent(s), will you have the resources (time, money, easy transportation) to keep up with visits?

8. What if contact with your child's birth parent(s) lessens or stops completely despite your best efforts? How would you explain the absences to your child?

9. Will you consider your child's birth mother part of your "family" and provide financial/emotional assistance when needed?

10. If your donor is a close friend, will you let your child know his biological connection with this person?

Scientifically speaking, maintaining a relationship with a donor or birth parent is uncharted territory. This much we do know: when possible, an open arrangement with a child's birth or donor parent is best for all involved. How open these relationships should be is still being studied. Obviously, time with a biological parent who is severely troubled must be limited, but deciding on what boundaries need to be placed should involve counselors and professionals that have advanced knowledge on the subject.

What difficult questions could you be asked by your adopted or donor child?

It's just a matter of time, but all parents of adopted or ART children get them: the zinger questions. Asked out of curiosity, and never due to a lack of love, all children develop a natural desire to know more about their genetic origins. Instead of dreading or ducking the questions, smart parents are prepared with intelligent and nurturing answers. Think of responses to the hard questions below. You may never be asked one or more of the questions, but isn't it better to have a practiced response ready?

1. Was my birth mother crazy or a drug addict?
2. Will I be a drug addict when I get older too?
3. Did my birth mother give me away because I was bad?
4. Was I stolen from my birth mother?
5. How much did I cost?
6. How do I know my birth mom isn't trying to find me?
7. Does my biological father know I exist?
8. Can you get a picture of my birth mom? If not, why?
9. Now that my birth mother is older, has more money; is married, etc., will she ask for me back?
10. Why doesn't my birth mother call?
11. If you could have your own baby, would you still have adopted me?
12. Why can't I have, curly hair, blue eyes, etc., like you?
13. Why didn't a Chinese (or nationality of your adopted child) family adopt me?
14. Will you be sad if I find my birth mother or if she finds me?
15. Am I being mean (or does it upset you) when I ask questions about my birth mother?

All children are curious about their origins. Discussing the birds and the bees with an adopted or ART-conceived child, however, adds a few more dimensions to the conversation. Ronny Diamond, CSW and Director of Spence-Chapin Adoption Resources, offers this suggestion in his article *Talking with Your Kids About Adoption:* "Answering the question 'Where do I come from?' involves discussions about birth, reproduction, and adoption. If your child doesn't ask, you can raise the topic yourself; find out what your child thinks and what he wants to know. It is better to respond to questions than to inundate a child with information."

CHAPTER 6

Bringing Home Your Baby

"We had lots of people at our house when we first brought our baby home. It was noisy, and crowded, but the baby didn't mind, he was all quiet and calm. As soon as the door closed when the last person left, Boom! He started screaming and didn't stop crying from 9:00 p.m. to 7:00 a.m. I looked at my wife and said, 'Oh-oh, here we go!'"

-Steve, father of two sons, ages 22 and 25 years

"When we got home from the hospital my husband and I looked at each other and thought, Oh, Sh#@t! What do we do now?"

-JP, mother of a 19-year-old son

You've survived the delivery, or if you're adopting, the "gotcha" moment, and you're ready to take your little miracle home. As you drive away from the hospital, you realize you're on your own. If your baby cries, breaks out in a rash, won't eat, or leaves some funky diaper deposits, it's up to you to figure out what to do next. Don't despair if it takes three attempts before you put the diaper on right, or if you can't tell the difference between hungry or tired crying. All parents go through a learning curve. Take the quiz below to find out your newborn-readiness.

Are you prepared to bring home a newborn?

1. What direction should an infant car seat face when properly installed?
    a) child facing back of car
    b) child facing front of car

2. Which of the following do newborns NOT need when given a bath
    a) soap
    b) a wash cloth or sponge

3. When should you give your baby her first bath in a tub?
    a) only after the umbilical cord stump has fallen off and the scar healed
    b) as soon as the infant is brought home from the hospital

4. Why shouldn't you have a big "Welcome Home" party for your newborn?
    a) people can unknowingly pass along germs and illnesses to your newborn
    b) seeing unfamiliar faces will scare your baby

5. The most common mistake new parents make when dressing their newborns is:
    a) overdressing their child during warm weather
    b) dressing their baby in clothes two sizes too large

6. What should you do if your newborn sleeps through the night her first night home?
    a) wake her up every four hours for a few weeks to prevent dehydration
    b) count your blessings

7. What's the best position to lay your baby down for a nap?

    a) on the baby's side, propped up with pillows

    b) on the baby's back

8. What are the five "S" words experts recommend to help calm your newborn?

    a) sit, sing, smile, be silly, or give sweets

    b) swing, swaddle, shush, side/stomach position, and sucking (feed or give pacifier)

9. How many diapers does the average newborn go through a day?

    a) 3-6 diapers

    b) 7-10 diapers

10. Between naps, how long do newborns usually stay awake?

    a) between two to four hours

    b) between 45 minutes to an hour

11. The two most important things to do before lifting your baby are:

    a) make sure your nails are short, you're securely holding the baby at the waist

    b) wash your hands and support the baby's head

12. Which is the correct technique to dislodge an item from a choking infant's throat?

    a) Heimlich maneuver

    b) back blows and chest thrusts

The correct answer for questions 1-6 is option "a." In addition to installing the infant car seat facing the back of the vehicle, do not use a car seat over two years old, or that has been in an accident, even if practically new. Bathing your newborn too early, or before the umbilical cord has completely healed, can cause irritation or an infection.

You should also avoid having your baby handled by too many people since humans are walking germ transmitters, especially during cold and flu season. As for the cute little sweater outfits, if it's too warm for you to bundle up, it's too much for your baby. Finally, although it sounds counterintuitive, it's important that a developing infant eat every few hours to avoid dehydration, even if it means interrupting your baby's sweet slumber.

The correct answer for questions 7-14 is option "b." Don't even think of setting an infant down near anything plush that could cause suffocation, and singing and smiling at your baby may warm your heart, but it probably won't quiet your fussy infant. According to Dr. Harvey Karp, author of the *Happiest Baby on the Block* book series, the "S" actions in option "b" are surefire methods of calming even a colicky infant.

Newborns soil many diapers in a day, but they also take very long naps which will allow time to get some laundry done. And finally, infants are too fragile to be lifted by the waist or to be given the Heimlich maneuver. Whoever handles your child should do so with utmost care.

How will you feed your newborn?

Who would have known that breast-feeding would become such an emotionally charged topic? Legions of women have banded together to tout the benefits of breast milk over formula and demand that "lactation centers" be created in work and public places.

Yes, breasts are great, but many new mothers are surprised to find that breast-feeding can be difficult to master, and, for a small percentage of women, that their bodies can't produce enough milk to adequately feed their baby. Women who choose not to breast-feed, or can't for whatever reason, don't necessary have to rely on formula. A cottage industry has developed that aims to provide the benefits of a mother's milk (not necessarily from the baby's own) to all infants. There are wet nurses who breast-feed children other than their own, and milk banks that collect, pasteurize, test, and then sell milk from screened donors, ready to supply the miracle elixir to those in need. If it takes a village to raise a child, there's an entire block devoted to making sure your infant is well-fed.

Take the quiz that follows to test your knowledge of some fascinating facts about breast milk and infant formula.

Infant Feeding Facts	**True**	**False**
Your baby's poop will change if you switch from breast-feeding to formula.	___	___
Babies rarely are allergic to breast milk, but can have an allergic reaction based on certain foods the mother has eaten.	___	___
The more you breast-feed or pump, the more milk your body will produce.	___	___
Breast milk can be stored in a freezer from four to six months.	___	___
Babies digest formula slower, so they can go longer between meals.	___	___

Babies who are breast-fed have a lower risk of developing asthma, certain infections, and becoming obese.

_____ _____

Blood or mucus in your baby's stool could mean your baby is allergic to the formula you're using.

_____ _____

Alcohol will be present in your breast milk if you have a drink right before feeding your baby.

_____ _____

Breast milk changes in chemical composition several times a day.

_____ _____

A woman burns about 500 extra calories a day producing breast milk.

_____ _____

Breast-feeding produces a calming chemical reaction in a mother's brain.

_____ _____

The uterus of a nursing mother will heal more quickly than that of a mother who does not breast-feed her baby.

_____ _____

Formula-feeding mothers can bond with their babies just as well as those who breast-feed.

_____ _____

Breast milk provides a baby with antibodies. Formula does not.

_____ _____

The FDA requires infant formula to contain at least 29 different vitamins and minerals.

_____ _____

Always nursing your baby from the same breast can make you lopsided.

_____ _____

The majority of women with breast implants can still breast-feed.

_____ _____

The World Health Organization recommends women breast-feed their babies for at least six months.

_____ _____

It may take weeks for a baby and the mother to get the hang of breast-feeding.

_____ _____

Fussiness during feedings is normal and doesn't necessarily mean your baby isn't getting enough milk.

_____ _____

The good news is that all of the statements above are true. A list of lactation consultants, organizations and other resources can be found on The International Lactation Consultants Association's excellent website, www.ILCA.org. It also provides links to websites offering nutrition advice for both baby and nursing mother. You can also ask your clinician for references to local groups and services that will help you provide the best nutrition for your newborn.

Should you vaccinate your child?

We tend to forget how science has practically eliminated numerous health concerns that for centuries were accepted tragedies in life. Not many generations ago, women could expect to lose at least one child to an infectious disease such as polio or measles. Vaccinations have made these losses an exception, not the norm. Yet today, despite overwhelming evidence supporting their safety, vaccinations have become controversial. If you're still unsure about vaccine safety or want to make immunizing your child as risk-free as possible, answering the following questions may help you clarify your thinking.

1. Would you choose to not vaccinate your child, just because a celebrity or person close to you believed vaccinations were unsafe or unnecessary?

2. If you are doing research on vaccinations will you rely solely on data off the Internet, or will you personally interview doctors and scientists and visit medical libraries to get your information?

3. If you're non-vaccinated child becomes sick with an illness routinely prevented by immunization, would you be liable for helping spread the disease to others, especially the elderly?

4. Would you be forced to take extra safety precautions such as isolating your child away from sick children, that wouldn't be necessary had your child been vaccinated?

5. Instead of refusing, will you ask to limit the number of shots your child receives in one visit?

6. Is there a way to schedule shots further apart than recommended without putting your child at risk?

7. Will you ask your child's pediatrician if there are any shots that you can postpone until your child is older or ready to go to school?

8. Will you only vaccinate your child if the ingredients in the shot have never been accused of being toxic to children?

9. Will you only allow multiple shots to be given to your child if there have been tests verifying the safety of combining the formulas?

10. Will you only vaccinate your child if there are tests to ensure your child isn't allergic to any of the substances contained in the vaccine?

How will you know if your baby needs to see a doctor?

Imagine you're changing your newborn's adorable tee shirt and notice a rash on her back. In a panic you wonder, "Is it serious? Will it go away on its own? Was it something she ate, touched, or wore?" You feel helpless and then kick yourself for not going to med school. It's common for infants to develop some odd and somewhat scary conditions while adjusting to their first year outside of the womb. Naturally, you'll want to know if the condition is serious.

Below is a list of symptoms and situations you may encounter when caring for your infant. Enter "yes" if you think the description is serious enough to warrant an emergency call to your baby's pediatrician, or "no" if you believe the condition is commonly seen during infant development and can be treated with time or infant medication from a local drug store.

Is it serious?	Yes	No
An acne-like rash on the face and scalp		
Tiny white bumps around nose, chin or other parts of face		
Spitting up (not projectile vomiting) between feedings		
Producing black or very dark green poop a few days after birth		
A body temperature between 99 to 100 degrees		
Occasional diarrhea		
Flaky, crusty skin on scalp or dandruff		
Mild sunburn		
Signs of a lazy eye		
A birthmark that was not fading		
Smiling infrequently		

Bad nasal congestion		
An accidental burn blister		
Chewing on a dirty pet toy		
Crying uncontrollably for more than one hour		

Startling as they may be, all of the above are common and not life-threatening conditions among newborns that normally don't require emergency medical attention. The purpose of this exercise to help new parents understand that a newborn's body does more than just grow, it adapts to the new environment, with all its dust, sunlight, and treated water, in ways that produce odd and sometimes scary symptoms. Nonetheless, trust your instincts and use common sense. If your baby has experienced or shown any of the signs above and appears to be in pain, look listless, or refuses to eat, seek medical attention immediately.

How will you know if you're recovering properly?

With all your attention focused on your baby, will you neglect yourself? Carrying and delivering a baby is quite an ordeal for the female body, so don't expect it to bounce back and be bikini ready right away. It takes weeks for the body parts affected to heal and months or more for other postpartum symptoms to subside. While your hormone levels and muscles are trying to find their way back to normal, you may experience some of the conditions listed below. Enter "yes" if you believe the symptom is a sign of something more serious and warrants an emergency call to your physician, or "no" if you believe it's a normal part of the recovery process, and can be treated with time or over-the-counter medication found at your local drug store.

Is it serious?	Yes	No
More than 3 or 4 days of vaginal bleeding		
Bruising around your vagina or c-section incision		
Bruising anywhere else on your body		
Problems or pain while urinating		
Bloodshot eyes		
Blurred vision		
Night sweats		
Light-headedness		
Recurring constipation		
No bowel movement in over 3 days		
Soreness around vagina		
General soreness and low-grade fever		
Bouts of depression		
Loss of appetite		
Sore breasts		

You may not experience any or all the symptoms above, but they are common during the first few months of postpartum healing. Rarely serious, they're usually temporary and can be treated at home with rest and over-the-counter medication. However, you should inform your clinician at your next scheduled appointment if you've experienced any of the above so she can stay updated on your recovery. If vomiting and a fever accompany any of the above, or you also have a chronic illness, seek medical attention immediately.

CHAPTER 7

Care Giving

Federal law states that new mothers (and fathers) may take up to 12 weeks of unpaid maternity leave from their employer to care for their new baby. But after that it's back to work, and parents must find someone else to watch their child while they're on the job. Even if you plan to be a stay-at-home parent (SAHP), you'll need a trusted care giver to babysit while you run errands, attend adult functions, or take a much-needed nap. Finding and keeping a reliable, talented, and affordable care giver could be the most stressful endeavor you take on as a parent. If you're lucky, you'll find an individual or organization that treats your child as if there's no other in the universe. Make the wrong decision, and you may end up feeling as if you're caring for two children instead of one.

Will you be your child's primary care giver?

"Something happened to me as soon as my daughter was born. I became a super psycho-paranoid freak. When she was a baby, I didn't want anyone to hold her, and I still don't leave her alone with someone when I'm not in the room. I so hope this is just a phase."

-Joanna, SAHP

Thinking about being a stay-at-home-parent? Generations ago, it was the norm for mothers. Today, it's seen as a choice for those who can manage their expenses on one income. Daddies have joined the roster of SAHPs (stay-at-home-parent), but staying at home full time to care for a child full time is not for everyone. The patience and selflessness required to meet constant demands make it more of a vocation than a job or career choice. It's also discouraging to hear recent polls announce that SAHMs (stay at home mothers) worry, feel sad and stressed more than mothers who are employed. Thankfully, a flip side indicates that more than half of these homies would still describe themselves as "thriving." But is being a SAHP right for you? To help you decide, ask yourself the questions below.

1. Do you welcome the routine of playing children's games, watching children's TV programs, and listening to kiddie music all day long, day after day?

2. Do you look forward to preparing breakfast, lunch, dinner, and snacks for your child and family day after day?

3. Do you want to receive hugs & kisses from your child any time of the day?

4. Does the thought of not having to get up, dress up, and go off to work hold appeal?

5. Would it kill you to not see your child reach milestones (first giggle, word, or step) because you were at work?

6. Will you gladly swap the chance to move up in your career to be a SAHP?

7. Do you love the thought of not being on a schedule, and only waking and eating based on your baby's desires?

8. Are you choosing to be a SAHP because you *want* to, not because you've been told it's the right thing to do?

9. Do you look forward to thinking up creative ways to spend each day with a child who will depend on you for entertainment?

10. Will you be very proactive in signing up for activities or mommy groups that get you out of the house to interact with other adults?

11. Would you start your own parenting group if you didn't find a group (or one you liked) nearby?

12. Are you open to blogging or joining online SAHP forums to give and receive advice plus emotional support while at home?

13. Will you set up some sort of relief schedule with your partner to take over all baby duties once he/she gets home?

14. Will you try to work from home while being a SAHP?

15. Psychologically, will it be easy giving up a regular paycheck to become a SAHP?

16. Will you feel comfortable relying on someone else's paycheck instead of your own?

17. Will saying you're a stay-at-home-parent make you feel just as proud as saying you're a full-time, working professional?

18. Do you agree that working with a difficult toddler is just as annoying as with a pain-in-the butt boss, but unquestionably preferred?

19. Will you *not* hesitate to ask for help if you start feeling unmotivated after weeks of a nap, feeding, diaper changing, and cleaning routine?

20. Do you agree that being a SAHP can be hard and thankless, but it is still the best job in the world?

If you've answered the majority of the questions above with an enthusiastic "Yes!" you may find being a SAHP is your true calling. As Shelly Loving of www.epinions.com explains, "The financial aspects of it have never been easy, but so far it's worth all the beans and rice, meat loaf, and the millions of free carnivals we've attended instead of going on vacations."

Will a friend or family member be providing day care?

> *"My dad used to take him one day a week, and literally plop the baby in the stroller and walk along the bluff, smoking a cigar, for hours. And then, he would take a nap, on the grass, with the baby still in the stroller, the sun blaring down on the baby's face, while holding on to one of the stroller's wheels. The baby could have fallen out of the top of the stroller, number one; number two, the baby came home sunburned on one side of his face. Then my dad would casually say, 'Oh, Nate got a little sun burnt today.' Then he'd go out a few days later and do the same thing again!"*
>
> -JP, mother of a 19-year-old son

Relatives and friends make up the majority of child care providers; grandparents alone watch 38 percent of all preschool aged children. Many parents feel more confident turning over their child to someone they've vetted through friendship or blood ties. Arranging for a relative to care for your child is usually less formal than employing professional help but should be considered with equal seriousness. Set up review meetings every few months to see if the arrangement still works for everyone involved or needs to be modified.

If you're planning to have your parents or in-laws watch your child, consider their present *and future* physical abilities. Your parents may seem spry and agile today, but could they keep up with your child as he ages or gains siblings? Be considerate of the other person's time and efforts. Never assume a parent or sister is available at your disposal because she "stays home all day anyway" or "has nothing better to do" in the afternoon. Watching your child may be more fun than a day at Disneyland, but all that joy takes a lot of energy and is at the expense of doing other activities.

In the questions below, "relative" can refer to a parent, in-law, sibling or other close relation.

1. Has your relative shown a strong, lukewarm, or indifferent or resigned interest in providing day care for your child?

2. Will you set up a regular schedule or expect your relative to watch your child on demand?

3. Will you reimburse your relative for any incidentals (emergency diaper runs, movie tickets, fast food lunches) they purchase while watching your child?

4. Will he/she be caring for your child in your home or theirs?

5. What will you do if your parents and in-laws are in a tug-of-war over who will babysit your child?

6. Will your relative provide day care because you frankly can't afford anyone else?

7. Will your relative have a long commute or travel late at night to be with your child?

8. Will caring for your child make it difficult for your relative to schedule doctor appointments or attend social functions?

9. Will watching your child keep your relative from helping another sibling with children?

10. If your parents will be providing day care, do you want them to treat your child exactly as you were treated growing up?

11. How are you going to adjust to the fact that as children age, their energy level goes up, but as your parents age their energy level goes down?

12. What would you do if your relative hinted or complained that your child was too much for them to handle?

13. Would you mind if your relative occasionally had a "substitute" watch your child?

14. What would you do if your relative completely ignored your house rules and other instructions you asked to be followed?

15. What would you do if your child were injured from an accident while being watched by your parents?

16. Does your relative have any physical or medical conditions such as poor eyesight, a bad back, or trouble lifting that could affect their child care abilities?

17. How would you react if you came home and found your relative snoozing while your toddler was roaming around the house alone?

18. Besides asking "Why?" what would you do if your child said they did not like spending time with the relative?

19. Will your relative be watching other children at the same time they care for your child?

20. If your relative is single, but dating, will you allow her or him to watch your child with a boyfriend or girlfriend?

21. What would you do if your relative became sick or injured and could no longer care for your child?

22. What would be a situation or event that would make you replace your relative as care givers?

23. Could you "fire" a care-providing relative? Would doing so cause long-lasting family resentments?

24. Will you give your relative full and unquestioned authority over your child?

25. Will you set limits or give specific, written instructions as to what your relative can and cannot do while watching your child?

Will you hire a professional care giver to help care for your child?

"The ideal situation is to not put too much pressure on your nanny. It stresses everyone out, even the children. I'm not saying parents have to be lax; they have to have some rules, but not be a slave to the rules. Nannies are just like any professional; we're humans that do our best without the added pressures."

-Cecilia, nanny caring for a 9-year-old boy and 12-year-old girl

"I went to get my hair colored, and during that morning several of my friends called the house. Our Austrian au pair told them I was out and that I went to the 'saloon' rather than the 'salon.' My friends called my cell one by one, asking what had happened that I needed a beer at 9:00 a.m."

-Mass Mom at AuPairMom.com

Having a professional care giver work with you is more than a luxury; it's welcoming another member into your family. Winston Churchill famously said of his nanny, "My nurse was my confidante. She had been my dearest and most intimate friend during the whole twenty years I had lived. I shall never know such a friend again." To underscore the value of this vocation, in some cities where parents compete for resources, a good nanny can easily out-earn a doctor.

Interested in hiring a full-time nanny?

1. Do you insist your care giver is a college graduate with advanced child care training?
2. Is it important that your child's care giver has been thoroughly screened by a nationally recognized service?
3. Are you willing to collect and pay payroll taxes and file the required tax forms as an employer?
4. Are you willing to pay a professional level salary, with benefits, to a qualified candidate?

If you answered "yes" to the questions above, you'll have no problem considering a full-time nanny, the gold standard for at-home child care. Nannies of all experience ranges can be found through agencies or freelance advertisements. There is no license designation for nannies, but there are agencies licensed by the state in which they work that screen applicants and only hire out individuals meeting certain strict criteria. Top-notch nannies are professionals that often hold a degree in some area of child development. Expensive and in demand, they can ask for and receive paid holidays, vacations, employee benefits, raises, and bonuses. For those who describe their nanny as an indispensable organizer, moderator, pacifier, facilitator, and overall miracle worker, it's money well spent.

Could an au pair be right for you?

1. Are you looking for full-time help at a lower cost than hiring a full-time nanny?
2. Do you expect to only need full-time assistance for a couple of years?
3. Do you like the idea of easily changing care givers as your child gets older?
4. Would you prefer a younger care giver that is less set in her care-giving ways?

If you've answered "yes" to the questions above, perhaps an au pair might be perfect for your family. Au pairs are foreign nationals between the ages of 18 and 26 years, trained to work abroad as an in-house child care provider under a special visa. They are hired through an approved agency to live, eat, and vacation with a family while providing child care for up to 45 hours a week. They don't do housework and cannot watch children unsupervised overnight. Au pairs stay with a family for a minimum of one and maximum of two years. They are less expensive than a nanny but have more restrictions and conditions to their employment.

Could a babysitter meet your care-giving needs?

1. Do you only need someone to watch your child for a few hours a day?

2. Will you only need a care giver sporadically or with little advance notice?

3. Could you see yourself hiring someone to accompany you on vacations or to events to help watch and care for your baby?

4. Do you feel you're just as good a judge of character and skill as an outside employment agency?

If you answered "yes" to the above questions, perhaps you'll be more than happy hiring a babysitter on an as-needed basis. Babysitting has come a long way since the days when parents would simply rely on the teenager next door. Sitter searching has gone high tech and moved up a couple of notches in the process. There are babysitter referral websites, online screening agencies, social network child care co-ops, and popular employment websites that list babysitters armed with college degrees, CPR certification, even fluency in sign language. Some sitters are available on short notice, but the more perks and professional services offered, the more you should expect to pay.

What should you consider when hiring a care giver?

"I hired a babysitter only once, when my son was a toddler. When my husband and I came home the babysitter was asleep on the sofa and our son was roaming around the house unsupervised. Couldn't she at least have stayed awake?"

-Heather, mother of a 7-year-old son

The Internet has made finding available care givers easier than ever. Parents can sift through various websites offering nannies suitable for royalty, au pairs fluent in the foreign language of your choice, or babysitters who are experienced with autistic children. Whether searching for a live-in nanny or occasional babysitter, knowing what you want ahead of time will help cut through a long list of able candidates. The questions below will give you a better picture of what qualities you think are most important when looking to hire a care giver and how thoroughly you're willing to vet the person you'll be welcoming into your home.

1. What's the number one qualification you'll be looking for when hiring a care giver?

2. Which of the following will you do on a candidate before offering them a job: credit check, background check, calling referrals, validating licenses?

3. Would you still do a background check if you were hiring a person recommended by someone close to you?

4. Will you ask to see a candidate's Facebook page or ask to review her online activities?

5. Would you only hire a care giver that came with several letters of recommendation?

6. Would you avoid hiring someone who was only working in child care as a means to fund schooling to start another type of career?

7. Would you hire a care giver that wasn't licensed or insured?

8. When hiring a care giver, how old is too old and how young is too young?

9. Will you rely on an agency to screen and recommend potential care givers?

10. Would you prefer or refuse to hire a male or female care giver?

11. Would you hire a care giver that was very physically attractive?

12. How much education do you expect your care giver to have?

13. What would be on your list of deal breakers when hiring a care giver?

14. How do you feel about hiring someone of a different race, culture, or religion?

15. Do you want a care giver who can teach your child a foreign language?

16. If a potential care giver spoke with a heavy accent, would you worry about her ability to be understood if she had to call 911?

17. What would you do if your partner disliked a care giver you really wanted to hire?

18. Under what conditions, if any, would you hire an undocumented immigrant as a care giver?

19. Could you trust your care giver to spend unsupervised time in your home with access to your valuables?

20. If you were desperate for a sitter to come on short notice, would you hire a stranger from an ad online?

Not too long ago, there was a popular photo of a baby and stuffed duckie carefully duct-taped to a wall making the rounds on the Internet. Fortunately, parents don't have to go to such extremes to keep an eye on their child. With websites such as www.sittercity.com and www.sitters.com parents can find excellent, reliable child care help at their fingertips.

What are the benefits of having a child care contract?

Professional child care workers will often present you with a detailed contract explaining their services and rate. If the person you're about to hire, be it a stranger or close friend, does not have or suggest a contract, draft one. Putting things down on paper goes a long way in avoiding future misunderstandings. Below are rules and regulations for care givers to follow while watching your child. Check the column to mark the ones that you feel are important enough to include in your contract.

While watching your child, will you allow your care giver to...	Yes	No
watch soap operas, Mature/PG-R rated TV shows or movies while your child is in the room?	_____	_____
text or call friends?	_____	_____
do homework or browse the web?	_____	_____
visit a friend with your child?	_____	_____
have visitors over to the house?	_____	_____
use the family car?	_____	_____
take food and drinks from your kitchen?	_____	_____
drink an alcoholic beverage?	_____	_____

	Yes	No
take naps?	_____	_____
leave your home with your child?	_____	_____
bring your child gifts, candy, or other snacks?	_____	_____
prepare snacks or meals at your home?	_____	_____
run personal errands with your child?	_____	_____
take pictures of your child?	_____	_____
punish your child with time-outs or other restrictions?	_____	_____
discuss religious themes or tell religious stories?	_____	_____
teach your child how to play poker or other gambling games?	_____	_____
play box, wrestle, or engage in other types of rough play your child?	_____	_____
bring their pet(s) to your home?	_____	_____
watch your child while sick with a cold or other minor illness?	_____	_____

Phone plans, gym memberships, and home renovators all have contracts, so it's incomprehensible to neglect having a contract with a person responsible for watching your most precious asset—your child. It's highly advisable to have a written agreement with a care giver that includes the stipulations made above along with pay rate, scheduled hours, benefits (if any), plus the duties you're expecting the person to perform while on the job.

What questions should you ask a prospective day care facility?

"I was ready to hire what I thought was the perfect day care provider until she let it slip that she didn't qualify to work at a public school because she tested positive for hepatitis."

- Carol, mother of 10-, 12- and 24-year-old sons

If you plan to enroll your child in a day care facility, you're not alone. According to the National Association of Child Care Resource and Referral Agencies (NACCRRA), 63 percent of America's children under the age of five regularly spend time in care centers outside their homes. Your area may offer several options such as for-profit, not-for-profit and co-op centers, employee associated services, and unlicensed day care providers.

Unlike pre-schools, which have a curriculum usually aimed at preparing children for kindergarten, a day care center's main objective is to care for your child in your absence. You've already touched upon the potential costs of day care in Chapter 2 and can apply many of the questions directed at choosing the right school found in the next chapter to finding a suitable day care facility. The questions below focus on your feelings about enrolling your child in an outside care center and how you expect to manage the costs.

1. Would you only feel secure sending your child to a day care center that was fully licensed?

2. Is it important that all certifications and licenses be visible or readily available for parents to review?

3. Would you leave your child in a facility that was unlicensed but had a great staff?

4. Does the facility encourage parents to drop in any time?

5. Will you feel guilty leaving your child in a day care facility?

6. Do you feel it's healthy for you and your child to spend some time apart?

7. Do you feel your child will get more mental stimulation at a day care center than at home?

8. Will you find it hard to trust any staff members at a day care center?

9. Do you feel uncomfortable having your child play with kids you've never met?

10. If your child started acting up would you blame the day care for teaching her bad habits?

11. Will you worry that your child will start liking day care more than spending time with you?

12. If your child gets sick, will you blame the day care for being unsanitary?

13. Would it be OK to send your child to day care with a slight case of the sniffles?

14. Will you ask relatives to help you pay for day care?

15. Will the cost of day care be more than what you earn from your job?

Although costs and logistics are often the primary reason a parent chooses a day care provider, the most important factor should be your confidence that you will be dropping off your child to a place that is second only to your own home in offering a caring and nurturing environment.

CHAPTER 8

Your Child's Education

"People stress too much about their kid's education in, I'd say, kindergarten through middle school. Let them enjoy themselves. Let them fall on their knees. Let them learn that they can't always get the teacher that they want. Don't fight for that teacher in third grade. Let loose in the formative years; don't let the kids see you stress about the teachers because then they'll be unhappy and stress out. If someone had said to me Donna, she doesn't have to have AP classes in ninth grade I would have hugged her today."

–Donna, mother of 20-year-old daughter attending UCLA

How can you help your child have future academic success?

With all the clamoring and stressing over whether or not a child should attend preschool or is getting into the right kindergarten, it's evident that parents overlook the single most important influence on how well their child will perform academically: their own involvement with their child's education.

Though there's no guarantee that playing Mozart while pregnant, or continuously reciting the alphabet to your expanding womb will have you produce a future Rhodes scholar, what you do choose to do with your child and how you do it will have a major impact on your child's academic performance. To see if you'll be interacting with your child in a way that promotes positive scholastic results, choose your most likely course of action between the options below.

Will you ...

start using flash cards to play with your child as soon as possible,	or	leave all that flash card playing to the kindergarten teacher?
enroll your child in preschool, despite the extra expense,	or	skip preschool. It's unnecessary or not worth the money?
give your child early music lessons,	or	let your child decide if she wants to sign up for music classes if the program is available in her school?
spend more hours reading and playing games,	or	watch TV with your child?
visit a library or a museum at least a few times a week,	or	only visit when scheduled as a school field trip?
make a progress chart to track your child's educational achievements,	or	leave the chart making and tracking up to the school; you have enough to do?
explain the benefits of doing well in school, but never offer a gift in exchange for a good grade,	or	bribe your child to do well in school?
spend more time encouraging and helping your child do well,	or	punish your child if she brought home a bad report card?

let your child know from day one that he is expected to get a college education,	*or*	do you feel college isn't for everyone, so you won't mention it to your child?
create a quiet and comfortable place for your child to do school projects and practice lessons,	*or*	expect her to do them in a room with distractions and discomforts?
set up a regularly scheduled time to do educational lessons or homework each day,	*or*	fit in lessons and homework help whenever you can find free time?
tell your child about wonderful teachers and how much fun you had in class when you were a kid,	*or*	admit that you hated school and were forced to go to class?
teach your child to respect her teachers,	*or*	frequently tell your child her teacher is wrong or doesn't know what she's talking about?
tell your child there's value in all lessons taught in class,	*or*	dismiss a lesson with the comment, "Don't worry, you'll never use this stuff in real life"?
allow your child's school schedule to take priority over any other obligations,	*or*	do you think it's OK to have your child skip school to help if you need help at home, or to take a day trip?
brush up on your own math skills or learn a new language along with your child to help with their education,	*or*	support but not get involved with your child's school lessons?

If you mostly chose the sentences on the left, you're moving in the right direction to help your child do well academically. According to recent studies, heavy-handed tactics like bribes, threats, and punishments may temporarily motivate a child to do well in school, but soon backfire once the fear or desire for the reward subsides. Indifference or irreverence toward anything academic-teachers, lessons, or higher education—usually makes a child feel that school isn't important, or that academic excellence isn't something he should aspire to achieve. Parents who present school and academics in a positive light and are involved in their child's homework and a school's programs, plus offer encouragement when their child is struggling, regularly see good scholastic results.

What should you consider when choosing a school for your child?

"The philosophy of the school room in one generation will be the philosophy of government in the next."

-Abraham Lincoln

It may seem very premature to be thinking about where your child will get his education when you haven't even started a baby registry, but it's important to gather information on your child's future school choices, since it is often the primary reason parents choose to stay in or leave a neighborhood. The school selection process has changed dramatically, moving way beyond deciding between a public or private education. In many communities, there's a dizzying array of choices in each system, making the distinction almost irrelevant. If your area offers several school options at various costs, you'll appreciate having the extra time to do your research.

To help you sift through the scholastic selections that await you, keeping your sanity intact, use the following barometer to find out your priorities when choosing a program. In short, what would you like the ideal school to offer?

Campus Criteria

Location and physical amenities

How important is it that the school...	Very	Somewhat	Not at all
is located close to your home or work?			
not be located next to a busy street or commercial center?			
provides convenient and safe bus service to class?			
allows parents to drop their kids off early?			
provides after school activities for children whose parents must pick up their kids late?			
has a good security system around the campus?			
has a big outdoor playground for running and playing sports?			
has computers and up-to-date equipment in the classroom?			
has a well-stocked library that is used often?			
is in a building that is new or recently updated and renovated?			

Faculty and staff

How important is it that...	Very	Somewhat	Not at all
the school only employs teachers and assistants with advanced degrees in education?			
the school has adequate staff to supervise playground activities?			
your child's teacher allows parents to help in the classroom?			
your child's teacher maintains a website that shows class assignments and scheduled events?			
your child's teacher is easily accessible by email or phone?			
the school has a low turnover of faculty and staff members?			
you personally like all of your child's teachers?			
the school's teachers rank highly on teacher rating websites?			
the school provides aides for students who are struggling or have special needs?			
the school has the lowest student-to-teacher ratio in your area?			

Teaching philosophies and methods

How important is it that the school...	Very	Somewhat	Not at all
has the highest academic rating in your area?			
spends more time on academic drills than play time or art projects?			
stresses individual learning, with students learning at their own pace (Montessori method)?			
follows a predictable routine that emphasizes creative learning within a group (Waldorf method)?			
promotes parent and student collaboration in class and with assignments (Reggio Emilia method)?			
has a bilingual program and includes lessons on other cultures?			
frequently schedules field trips to museums or other teaching environments?			
serves healthy lunches and promotes an eco-friendly campus?			
teaches music?			
not allow activities related to religious beliefs (Christmas pageant, prayer in class)?			

Classmates

How important is it that...	Very	Somewhat	Not at all
your child enrolls in the same school that most neighborhood kids attend?			
the school has a diverse student population?			
you avoid a school where many of the students and their parents don't speak English?			
the school is a single sex (all boy or girl) campus?			
your child's classmates come from families that are just as wealthy as or wealthier than yours?			
the school has a "no-tolerance" policy toward bullying?			
the school has a policy of sending home sick and contagious children?			
there be a high degree of gifted students in your child's class?			
the school has a low incidence of playground fights?			
children are not brought in from outlying neighborhoods?			

What type of school would be the best fit for your family?

With the developments of magnet and charter schools in the public education system, the line between public vs. private education has been blurred. Students in private schools no longer are the guaranteed better performers over their public counterparts, and public schools can be run independent of government boards and bureaucracy, a privilege once only enjoyed by private institutions.

With these distinctions gone, the decision as to whether to go public, private, or to turn your own house into a school by homeschooling your child usually comes down to dollars and cents or personal preference.

Would you prefer to enroll your child in a public school?

"The benefit of sending your child to a public school is the technology. You can monitor, research, and find out all sorts of information on the school online. I mean, teachers can only tell you so much. I like www. greatschools.org. With all these wonderful tools, why not use what our tax dollars support?"

-Carol, mother of sons ages 25, 12, and 10 years old.

1. Do you believe it's important to support the public education system?
2. Would you agree with the statement, "I've already paid for the school with my taxes, so why go elsewhere?"
3. Does the performance of your local public school rate higher than that of a neighboring private school?

4. Will you feel more involved with your community by sending your child to a public school?

5. Does your neighborhood offer magnet or charter schools that are highly rated?

6. Does your public school have a strong program for children with special needs should your child require specialized help?

If you answered "yes" to a majority of the questions above, then a public school may be the perfect fit for your family. Although by law public schools must accept all children, popular schools with programs for the gifted or those with learning disabilities may base admission on lottery results, waiting lists, or an involved application process. This underscores the importance of beginning your research early so you're aware of submission requirements and deadlines.

Would you prefer to enroll your child in a private school?

"My husband said he was impressed with my values and assumed I learned them from my years of private, Catholic schooling, so that's what he wanted for my daughters. I brought up the costs, but they were never a concern for him, because it was so important to him to have them go private. In retrospect, I'm glad he insisted. It has made my daughter a stronger person. She had major separation anxiety in kindergarten. The teachers and a group of students got together to make sure she was taken care of. She learned that it was OK to meet all these people, because they'll take care of you. I don't think she would have gotten that in public

school because they don't have enough resources to focus on one student, and the teachers, because of more restrictions, have limits on how they can interact one-to-one. My daughter would have been more guarded, because they (the teachers) have to be guarded."

-Tiffany, mother of 5- and 9-year-old daughters

To some, the title of private school conjures up images of nuns with rulers or preppy children in uniforms. Perhaps there are schools that fit that mold, but not all of them do. There are nonreligious schools that focus on different learning theories and methods, place emphasis on the arts, or work exclusively with children with disabilities. Private schools are the obvious choice for parents who have a specific theme they want their child's school to follow. The questions below will help you determine whether your requirements will be best served by a school that is privately funded and managed.

1. Do you want a school that specifically emphasizes the arts or sciences?
2. Do you want a school that offers religious as well as academic instruction?
3. Do you want a school that offers the smallest class size in your area?
4. Are you comfortable participating in frequent fund drives and charity auctions?
5. Are the public schools managed poorly or rate substantially lower academically than the private schools in your area?

If you answered "yes" to the questions above, a private school may be in your child's future. Frequently parents cite costs as the biggest obstacle to sending their child to a desired private school. Yet many institutions provide ample financial aid or are tuition free. Parents also cite poor public school performance as a top reason for choosing to go private. If that's the buzz around your neighborhood, check out the public school for yourself. Many areas have been able to turn their schools around or have introduced charter campuses which have excellent teachers and strong learning programs. Bottom line: don't make your decision purely on rumors. The tuition you may save during your child's early schooling could go toward funding a college education in the future.

Would you prefer to homeschool your child?

"What does it take for someone to homeschool? Dedication and time. Dedication means having the willingness to look for what works best for you and your child, while recognizing both of your unique abilities. Then taking the time to apply your choices, and reassess as needed. What a home educator must often remember in the beginning is that we are the experts of our children. So, while the ways I home educate might not sound great to one parent, it might be just what this other parent is looking for."

-Rocio, mother of a 15-year-old, homeschooled
daughter and a 24-year-old son

For many of the same reasons some parents choose to enroll their child in a private school, (better environment, religious instruction), a growing number of parents will opt to educate their child at home. The abundance of academic materials, lesson plans, homeschooling co-ops and support groups available show that there's plenty of resources to feed the demand. To see if you may be up to the challenge of homeschooling your child, answer the questions below:

1. Are you willing to devote a good chunk of your time to creating lesson plans and arranging educational field trips for your child?

2. Do you have the resources to buy school supplies, instructional materials, and pay for museum visits or other events?

3. Are there other homeschooled children in the neighborhood with whom you could arrange group projects, games, or social functions?

4. Will you regularly attend educational conferences to constantly update and enhance your teaching skills?

5. Will you hire tutors or find others to instruct your child in subjects you don't feel you can teach well?

If you answered "yes" to the questions above, you may have what it takes to become the headmaster or mistress of your own home classroom. The costs and time required to homeschool takes some parents aback, but most admit it's worth the effort. If only for a few years, the ability to have full control of your child's academic progress and work one–on-one with your child can be priceless.

An area's school availability varies greatly across the country. It's not uncommon for less-populated areas to only have one school that all the children in the surrounding areas attend. Big cities, on the other hand, have so many options that parents find themselves frantically applying to various schools and academies hoping to land a spot in one of many coveted campuses. If you find yourself debating between two or more schools, the comparison table below can help you make a selection.

School Comparison Chart

Which school is or has the …	School A	School B	School C
Most economical?			
Most logistically friendly?			
Best security and safest?			
Highest academic standing?			
Nicest campus and best-kept facilities?			
Best student-teacher ratio?			
Most involved parents?			
Highest rated teachers?			
Most attended by children in the neighborhood?			
Preferred teaching method?			
Best after school programs?			
Most special needs programs?			

	School A	School B	School C
Most likeable staff?			
Preferred homework load?			
Preferred student conduct rules and enforcement?			
All-day care?			
Total points			

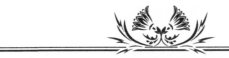

School Sign-up Checklist

Do you have the following ready to enroll your child in school?

☐ Birth certificate and/or baptismal record.

☐ Proof of residence (utility bill, voter registration, notarized statement).

☐ Record of your child's immunizations.

☐ Photo of your child for identification.

☐ List of your child's allergies or medical conditions (if any).

☐ List of emergency contact names and phone numbers.

☐ Names and an identifying photograph of people approved to pick up your child from school.

☐ Your and your child's social security number.

☐ Pay stubs or tax return showing eligibility for school lunch programs (if you qualify).

☐ Evidence that your child does not need eyeglasses or a hearing aid to properly see and hear his/her teacher during class.

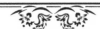

CHAPTER 9

Identity & Integrity

"For me, role models are real people in my life who I actually know. I think the girls, they're finding that the people in their lives—their dad, their niece, their cousins, my brother's kids—they look up to. I find kids are looking right in front of them. They don't view some old person in a book as a role model."

–United States First Lady, Michelle Obama

It will quickly become apparent that your child has his or her own mind, and personality. They're not a block of clay you can mold exactly to your specifications. Michelangelo once said of his famous sculpture, David, "I saw the angel in the marble and carved until I set him free." Time and experience will be the hammer and chisel that will release your child's individuality. Like the artist, a parent's role is to sand the rough edges, repair any cracks, and add polish so the final product can shine.

What tools will you use to buff your child into a confident, moral, and well-mannered child? Will you try to influence your child based on their gender, ethnicity, or your own philosophies?

Will you treat your child differently based on his or her gender?

"Do I treat my son and my daughter differently? Of course! Who doesn't? I think between a boy and a girl, you have different bonds and love for them, not that you love one more than the other–they're both very special. But, I'm way softer on my son. With my daughter I have less patience. I don't know why, I don't think I'm as tough with my son, but my husband is tougher on him than he is on my daughter. Maybe it's universal? I'm definitely drawn to the things I do with my daughter more, because she's a girl. But, I think with the mother-son relationship, you want them to look at you, or you think they look at you like the woman they want to be with later."

–Jami, mother to a 7-year-old son and 4-year-old daughter

Will you be a softy with a son, but dictator with a daughter? It's all so easy to say you'll be gender neutral, but what if your daughter recoiled at the sight of a princess doll or your son pined for a tea set instead of a Tonka truck? Toy preferences may be easy to dismiss, but what if you planned on bonding over traditionally sex-specific rituals like braiding your daughter's hair, or teaching your son how to bat? Even if you manage those situations well at home, will you continue to back your child's desires if they result in your child being teased relentlessly at school?

To see if your child's gender will make a difference on your behavior, put a check in the box that best matches what you'll allow based on your child's sex.

Would you...	Yes, if a boy	Yes, if a girl	No, if a boy	No, if a girl
give your child toy guns or other toy weapons to play with?				
mind if your child watches princess fairy-tale movies?				
mind if your child played dress up in mommy's clothes?				
mind if your child played dress up in daddy's clothes?				
gladly have your child join a hockey team?				
be bothered if a friend gave your child a cupcake decorating kit as a gift?				
teach your child how to sew or knit?				
enroll your child in a tap dance class?				
scold your child for hitting a girl?				
scold your child for hitting a boy?				
discourage your child from playing combat-intensive video games?				
mind if your child wanted glitter and feathers on outfits?				
let your toddler swim naked in public?				
allow overnight stays at a same-sex classmate's house?				

Would you...	Yes, if a boy	Yes, if a girl	No, if a boy	No, if a girl
allow overnight stays at an opposite-sex classmate's house (with parent supervision, of course)?				
sign up your child for Tae Kwan Do classes to see if he/she liked the sport?				
give your child growth hormones if the pediatrician determined he/she was likely to grow to be only 5' tall?'				
raise your child to be very rugged and outdoorsy?				
dress your child for a party in clothes that restricted his/her ability to climb trees or play sports?				
stop your child when he/she play wrestles with a friend or sibling?				
tell your child it's OK to cry when he/she falls down or is afraid?				
allow your child to be more rambunctious than a child of the opposite sex?				

Gender-neutral child rearing may be the ideal, but it's difficult to accomplish—try buying products for your daughter in something other than pink or purple. Perpetuating sexual stereotypes is more about suppressing or encouraging behaviors your child begins to show than scrutinizing where you shop.

How will you foster your child's racial and cultural identity?

"Public school is a melting pot, so it's easy to lose your culture. We're not religious, but I send my kids to Hebrew School. It's important to know who you are, and where you came from. I can't fathom my children not knowing that their great-grandparents were Holocaust survivors, or that this part of history didn't happen."

–Dorit, mother of 3-, 9-, and 11-year-old sons

You may feel race and culture are inextricably intertwined, engrained in your DNA, and passed on to your child along with your chromosomes. Perhaps you simply want to maintain certain cultural traditions regardless of the geographical, generational, or even ethnic changes your budding branch of the family may bring. Will you pass along the behaviors and beliefs of the culture you grew up with or have adopted as an adult? To get an idea how important this is to you, ask yourself the following questions:

1. What cultural traditions do you hope to pass on to your child?

2. Will you be reviewing cultural traditions you grew up with and deciding which you'll choose to pass on to your child and which you'll disregard?

3. Are there cultural traditions that your immediate family follows, but you don't want your child to participate in?

4. Do you feel it's important for a child to learn about the culture of his/her ancestors?

5. If your child is a melting pot of several nationalities, is it important that he/she learn about all the cultures or just selected ones?

6. Would you prefer that your child develop his/her own cultural identity based on his/her own generation, location, and personal experiences?

7. Will you continue to practice your culture's superior treatment of sons over daughters, or eldest son over all other siblings?

8. Is there a cultural practice you don't like but will follow to keep peace with other family members or peers?

9. If biracial, how would you feel if your child related more to only one side of his racial makeup?

10. How would you feel if your child had no interest or tried to distance him/herself from part of his cultural or racial heritage?

Don't be dismayed if your child doesn't show an interest in the cultural traditions you hold dear. Appreciation may come later in life. Renowned developmental psychiatrist Jean S. Phinney believes a person's ethnic identity comes in stages. Children accept the cultural norms taught by their parents without question. As they mature into adolescents and then young adults, they question and compare these beliefs and traditions, ultimately establishing a confident cultural perspective and ethnic identity.

What role will religion and spirituality play in your child's upbringing?

"It was our son that inspired us to become more spiritual. In the 5ᵗʰ grade, he chose to be baptized at our local church, and he really took it to heart. He felt a calling to follow a spiritual path. He never preached to us, nor his brother or sister, but his behavior was so positive and welcoming it drew us all to him and his beliefs. His (if you don't mind I'm keeping all children anonymous) strong, early commitment just exponentially increased our involvement and commitment."

–John & Patrice, parents of 24- and 21- year-old sons
and an 18-year-old daughter

There is a popular trend toward letting a child decide for himself what role religion will play in his life, but this decision will not happen in a vacuum. How parents express their opinions about church attendance, various denominations, and doctrine will be absorbed by their child and incorporated in his or her decision making process.

For parents who wish to pass on their faith to their children, there will be plenty of opportunities for teachable moments as children are naturally curious about God, angels, heaven, and other ethereal subjects. Spirituality can also be fostered without subscribing to a specific religion, for those parents who aren't comfortable with organized religion.

Faith and spirituality, whether inspired by the Bible, Koran, or nature, allow a child to trust things they can't yet understand and establish a sense of purpose for doing good and making positive, ethical choices. Being certain of your own spiritual beliefs will help you answer your child's inevitable theological questions, and living your life according to these convictions will guide your child to understand how theology is not just prayers and symbols, but a way of life.

Answer the questions below to clarify the spiritual philosophies you will pass on to your child:

1. How important is it that your child follows a specific religion?
2. At what age (if at all) will you begin giving your child formal religious instruction?
3. What compromises will you make when teaching religion to your child if you and your partner are of different faiths?
4. If you currently don't belong to a religious community, will you go "church shopping" to make religion a part of your child's upbringing?
5. Do you think it's acceptable to participate in religious rituals (baptism, bar mitzvahs) but not attend the religion's weekly services on a regular basis?
6. Will you encourage your child to only socialize with children of the religion you follow?
7. If you don't want your child raised with religion, how will you explain questions they will have regarding life after death, God, and religiously based holidays such as Easter?
8. Will you promote spirituality (prayer, love, and respect for all things living) but not endorse a formal religion?
9. If you want your child to discover religion on his/her own, will you object should he or she join a cult or faith you don't like later on in life?
10. If your child received an invitation to a church function from a friend of a different religion, would you allow him or her to attend?

A reverence and love for a higher being has been the catalyst for an immense amount of good as well as bad throughout humankind's history. We owe it to our children, ourselves, and the entire world to only use religion as a promoter of love, tolerance, forgiveness, and respect. Using religion to teach a child to hate, judge, or dismiss others is contrary to the values of practically every religious tenet.

How will you teach your child to be honest?

Your rules will be clear: lying is bad, and if you're like any good, fear-inducing parent, you'll throw in the gory story of *The Little Boy Who Cried Wolf* to bring home the point to your child. As you flail your arms and mimic screams for added effect, you'll be called to the phone. Without missing a beat, you'll reply, "Tell them I'm not home." Is it OK to tell a little white lie when you're trying to teach your child to be honest?

Following are some of the most popular little white lies and social deceptions parents often say or do. You may have heard a few from your own parents in your younger years, but which ones will you repeat to your child?

Which of the following will you say to your child?

	Acceptable	Avoid
"If you swallow the seeds, a vine will grow from your stomach."	_____	_____
"Santa, the Tooth Fairy, the Easter Bunny, etc., gives gifts to good boys and girls."	_____	_____
"Sesame Street isn't on today. The TV is broken."	_____	_____
"Your dolls ran away because you left them all over the floor."	_____	_____
"If you don't behave that police officer will arrest you."	_____	_____
"You'll catch a cold if you don't put on a sweater."	_____	_____
"We're all out of cake and cookies." (You hid them for yourself.)	_____	_____
"If you suck your thumb or play with your privates, they'll fall off."	_____	_____
"Your teeth will fall out if you eat that piece of candy."	_____	_____
"If you make a wish and blow out the candles, it will come true."	_____	_____
"A little bird told me you broke the vase."	_____	_____
"When the ice cream truck plays music it means they've sold out of ice cream."	_____	_____

George Bernard Shaw once said, "We must make the world an honest place before teaching our children that honesty is the best policy." Could you be teaching your child to be dishonest by answering "yes" to the questions that follow?

Will you...

1. lie about your child's age to get cheaper tickets?

2. tell your child that if the referee doesn't see him break the rules it doesn't count?

3. tell a teacher your child missed class because she was sick, when you really went to visit relatives?

4. fail to return a candy bar your child stole from a store because you're too tired to drive back?

5. sneak food into the movies instead of buying snacks at the theater's concession stand?

The occasional white lie told because the truth is not age appropriate (describing your brother's mistress as a "friend") or too upsetting (saying "fluffy went to live on a farm" when the dog was killed by a speeding car) is acceptable. Most often, parents and children are better served by turning the truth into a teachable moment, for example saying "Picking up a frog can hurt the animal" instead of perpetuating the myth that touching a frog causes warts. Liberally tossing out the white lies or worse yet, being dishonest in front of your child for personal gain, will send a clear message that lying is OK, especially if you benefit in the end. The best way to promote truthfulness in your child is to praise honesty, even when you don't like the answer ("Yes, Mommy, I spilled cocoa on the white rug"), and to act honestly, even when it's not the easiest thing to do.

How will you teach child to be fair and just?

As an adult, you're fully aware of the terrible inequality and injustices placed upon people by ruthless dictators or heartless governments. But to your child, there's no greater injustice than not being allowed to have ice cream for dinner, and it doesn't end there. She'll see others get larger slices of pizza and have toys taken away at dinner time—all too much for her little heart to bear. To prepare yourself for the inevitable call to be your child's judge, jury, and peacekeeping ambassador, practice giving responses to your child's complaints below.

What will you do when your child says:

"It's not fair! Why...

1. does he get a bigger piece of cake than me?"

2. does she get to cut in line when I was here first?"

3. does she get to wear nail polish and not me?"

4. did he get a new bike for Christmas and not me?"

5. didn't the teacher punish him for breaking my toy?"

6. wasn't I invited to her party?"

7. am I being punished when I didn't start the fight?"

8. can't I play 'Death & Dismemberment' (a game you've banned) like all my friends?"

9. didn't I get to be on the team?"

10. do I have to go to church when Dad gets to stay home?"

Teaching justice in an unjust world is difficult enough, but could you be showing your child that tipping the scales is acceptable behavior by responding "yes" to any of the questions below?

Will you...

1. cheer for TV characters that flaunt rules or are celebrated for breaking the law?

2. cut to the front of the line because the employee at the counter is your friend and will allow it?

3. punish your child for being late to dinner, even though you're chronically late for appointments and functions?

4. insist on special treatment at events or restaurants by saying, "Don't you know who I am?"

5. make comments that certain groups of people don't deserve the same rights as native citizens?

Being fair and just means more than same-sized servings and not taking an extra turn in checkers. It's a parent's responsibility to be fair but to also teach their child to know the difference between bigotry (not being able to join a team because of your religious beliefs) and bad luck (being denied because you missed the cut off date). You'll be your child's example of when to speak up against injustice and how to gracefully accept those times when luck isn't on your side.

How will you teach your child to be responsible?

Personal responsibility means cleaning up after yourself, completing chores, and being able to keep emotional outbursts under control. You probably don't know many adults that fit that description, so how can you instill those rare qualities into your child? A great technique is to assign tasks and responsibilities as soon as he/she is mature enough and physically able to carry them out.

How many chores will you put on your child's to-do list to make sure he learns the valuable trait of self-reliance? To get an idea, place a Y next to the chores you'll be assigning to your child, and the age you believe he/she should be before taking on the responsibility.

	Assign	Age
Put away toys after playing with them or at the end of the day	_____	_____
Clean his room by himself	_____	_____
Bathe himself and brush his teeth	_____	_____
Water plants	_____	_____
Put clothes in hamper or put away laundry	_____	_____
Clear or help set dinner table	_____	_____
Make his own bed	_____	_____
Feed a pet	_____	_____
Clean up any spills he causes	_____	_____
Pick out his own clothes and dress himself	_____	_____

Yes, you want your child to be responsible and self-reliant, but could you be teaching your child to be irresponsible by…

1. leaving your own clothes all over the floor or piled on top of furniture?

2. complaining daily about not being able to stay on a diet, quit smoking, or save any money?

3. regularly blaming others for failures or mistakes?

4. going ballistic while watching your team lose a game on TV?

5. allowing plants to die because of your forgetfulness or neglect?

Equally important as assigning the chores, it's imperative that parents be patient while their child masters the skills to do the job well. Mistakes will be made, and things may not be done perfectly, but your child will benefit from seeing his own improvement with time and age. Putting down your child's efforts is one way to discourage personal responsibility; another is to send mixed messages. How can a parent expect their child to be accountable when they can't be a good example?

How will you teach your child to show respect?

Respect is not unchallenged obedience; it's an expression of reverence for the integrity of objects and all things living. Manners are an outward sign of honor and empathy. Which manners you choose to have your child follow will probably be based on your culture and personal preference. Instruction can begin as soon as a child starts to talk and, according to grandmothers everywhere, should be re-taught to their adult children frequently.

Which of the following will you require from your child?

	Required	On occasion	Unnecessary
When with adults and authority:			
Use "Excuse me," "Please," "Thank you," and "You're welcome"	_____	_____	_____
Address adults as "Ma'am" or "Sir"	_____	_____	_____
No speaking unless spoken to	_____	_____	_____
Give up his/her seat to an adult	_____	_____	_____
Never to talk back to an adult	_____	_____	_____
No texting while being spoken to	_____	_____	_____
While at the dinner table:			
Wait for everyone to be seated and served before eating	_____	_____	_____
Eat with mouth closed, and don't talk while eating	_____	_____	_____
No eating off the plates of others	_____	_____	_____
Eat everything on the plate	_____	_____	_____
Leave a "courtesy" bit of food on plate	_____	_____	_____
Refrain from reading, texting, or bringing toys to the table	_____	_____	_____
Only leave the table when excused	_____	_____	_____

While playing sports or games with others:

No hogging the ball or taking turns
out of order

_____   _____   _____

No bragging when winning

_____   _____   _____

No whining, crying, or complaining
when losing a game

_____   _____   _____

Play by the rules

_____   _____   _____

Congratulate the winner

_____   _____   _____

Thank coaches or referees

_____   _____   _____

...with animals and the child's own personal property:

No damaging or destroying own toys

_____   _____   _____

Return borrowed toys in
good condition

_____   _____   _____

No cruelty (burning insects, pouring
salt on snails, etc.) to any animal
or insect

_____   _____   _____

No hitting or tormenting pets

_____   _____   _____

Good manners are an excellent way to have children show respect, but if parents don't explain that their purpose is to honor the feelings, property, and social standing of others, they are merely empty gestures.

Despite your best efforts, could you be teaching your child to be disrespectful by...

1. frequently making comments that the police, teachers, or coaches are idiots?

2. loudly complaining about the food you're served at home or in a restaurant?

3. talking loudly during movies, while in the library, or other places where silence is requested?

4. regularly insulting or talking back to your own parents even though you won't tolerate the same behavior from your child?

5. writing in library books or tearing pages out of communal magazines?

Ironically, parents often exclude themselves from the group of people that deserve deference by allowing themselves to be hit, yelled at, or ignored by their own children. Encouraging a child to question authority when they reach the age of critical thinking is fine; allowing them to insult or ridicule any person of authority should not be tolerated.

How can you teach your child to be compassionate?

Teaching children the golden rule surpasses showing them not to hit fellow classmates or to say "Sorry" when they do. Doing random acts of kindness and generosity helps teach a child that the world does not revolve around him/her and that altruism is the hallmark of a civil society.

Children have an innate capacity to show love and kindness, although you'll swear it doesn't exist while you're enduring your toddler's "me, me and mine, mine" stage. It's common, as the years go by and the demands to achieve increase, that practicing acts of compassion seem to fall by the wayside. Parents, however, shouldn't falter. As the Dalai Lama once said, "If you want others to be happy, practice compassion. If you want to be happy, practice compassion."

To teach your child compassion, will you ask your child to...

1. choose some of her toys to donate to the needy?
2. create care packages for those in need?
3. volunteer at a food bank?
4. help environmental group with clean-up or preservation project?
5. invite friends from other cultures to your home?
6. openly forgive someone who may have hurt his or her feelings?
7. visit someone in the hospital?
8. apologize if they make another child cry or take away their toy?
9. protect a child (by notifying a teacher) who is being bullied?
10. share her toys with other children?

Compassion in young children has to be cultivated by setting a good example and encouraging benevolence. Could you be teaching your child to be unkind by...

1. laughing when your child makes fun of any disabled children in his class?
2. regularly yelling and hanging up on people during phone conversations?
3. saying that giving money to panhandlers only supports their drug habit?
4. commenting that people on welfare or unemployment benefits are really just lazy and don't want to work?
5. making disparaging remarks about the children who receive government aid (free lunches, vouchers, etc.) at your child's school?

Let's be honest, financial or material displays of charity, writing a check, or giving away clothes that you no longer want are far easier than humbling yourself for the sake of others. If you think volunteering to work a shift at a soup kitchen with your child but then talking trash about mothers using food stamps to feed their families will teach your child compassion, think again. A parent's goal should be to create a compassionate child, not to collect check marks on a list of benevolent behaviors.

CHAPTER 10

Discipline

"Yelling doesn't work. We found that out real quickly. Anger only escalates things and gets you both more upset. I would say that once you find out what they like the most, you then use that as a reward for doing as they are asked, and doing their share; i.e., keep their room clean, etc. Simply holding objects back as a punishment gets them more upset, so it's best worded more like 'Let's just pick this stuff up quick and then you can get back to playing.' Boundaries need to be set and they will be respected... most of the time. It's always work in progress, requiring maintenance.

-Brian, father to four boys, ages 7- to 15-years-old

What type of disciplinarian will you be?

What if children could be trained like puppies? Potty training would be over after a few weeks of simply leaving your child on a toilet right after a meal. The loud slapping of a rolled-up newspaper on a nearby counter would quickly teach a teething child not to chew on the furniture, and with repeated praise and affection, you could teach a child to "stay" on command while you shop or leave a room without having to worry about what they may get into. Of course, this sounds ridiculous; children are not pets, but if you want results with either, discipline must be applied. How should this be done?

Below are four parenting styles. To find out which best describes how you'll be disciplining your child, circle the group that includes the most statements that you agree with or whose methods you're most likely to follow.

Type A Parenting:

Do you agree that...

1) children should be taught not to think but to obey?

2) a strict (but not cruel) military form of discipline is the most effective way to build a strong character?

3) parents who spend time negotiating with their kids are not teaching them to respect authority?

4) the phrases "My house, my rules," "Because I said so," or "When you pay the bills you can decide" are effective affirmation of a parent's authority?

5) if a child can't follow the rules and be at the dinner table at 5:30, they shouldn't be allowed to eat at the table?

Type B Parenting:

Do you agree that...

1) parents should discuss punishment options with their child?

2) if a child breaks a house rule, they should be given a chance to explain themselves before being punished?

3) explaining why something is wrong is more important than enforcing punishments?

4) discipline techniques should not impose on your child's self-esteem?

5) dinner time is flexible and can be whenever everyone can come together to eat?

Type C Parenting:

Do you agree that...

1) children learn best through their own trial and error?

2) strict parenting causes kids to rebel and get into trouble?

3) parents should strive to be their child's best friend instead of an overbearing disciplinarian?

4) your own parents were lenient, but you turned out fine?

5) dinner time will be whenever your child is ready to sit down and eat?

Type D Parenting:

Do you agree that...

1) someone else will primarily discipline your child because of your demanding work schedule?

2) children are resourceful and can learn to take care of themselves early on?

3) unless your child is in danger, it's not necessary to scold or punish him?

4) disciplining a child just teaches them to misbehave behind your back or in secret?

5) someone else will be preparing meals for your child, since you won't be home for dinner?

If the stern, whip-cracking method of parenting described by style A appeals to you, the type of discipline you lean toward is authoritarian. You set firm rules and expect them to be followed with minimum questioning. There's no doubt that you'll love your child, but you will insist they know who is boss and follow your directives accordingly.

If you agreed most with the statements in Type B, you'll be an authoritative parent. You believe in explaining and exposing causes and consequences over quick punishment. Although most behaviorists favor this style, overdo the explaining and your child will likely tune out your long lectures.

If the statements in Type C are more your style, you'll be a permissive parent. You don't believe in sweating the small stuff, and feel (or hope) that your child will figure out right from wrong with experience and age. Maybe you're lenient because your goal is to be your child's best friend, and fear that enforcing punishments and putting limits on behaviors will cause your child to dislike you.

If circumstances put you squarely in the Type D style of parenting, you run the risk of being an uninvolved or "accidental" parent. Busy with other obligations or interests, you avoid or are physically away from the kiddie/parent drama part of disciplining your child. You have rules, but leave enforcing them to others.

Although you may lean strongly toward one style, most parents are a combination of two or more; for example, authoritarian about academics, and permissive about chores. Whichever methods you put into play, relying on the same tactics from your upbringing because you feel "That's how I was raised and I turned out OK" is a cop-out. Being a good disciplinarian is an acquired skill that constantly needs to be evaluated and honed. This means keeping up on the latest child-rearing research and understanding that a technique that may have worked on you may not work for your child.

You'll have rough days, that's for sure, but no parent is perfect. If it's any comfort, the one trait all types of parents share is the fear that they're too harsh or not harsh enough when enforcing their rules. With love in your heart and the best intentions, you can only try your best.

What disciplinary techniques will you use on your child?

> *"The hardest thing we've ever done is let our son cry himself to sleep. I literally had to hold my wife down so she wouldn't open the door and let him into our bed. The first night he fell asleep leaning on our door, the second night he cried a little, then it was over. Bedtime had always been an ordeal and finally, we had peace and quiet. I asked my wife 'Why didn't we do this two years ago?!'"*

-Steve father of 22- and 25-year-old sons

After identifying the best parenting style, you need to investigate the best disciplinary techniques to apply when your child misbehaves. You're familiar with time-outs, and taking away TV privileges, but what's the most effective way to use these and other disciplinary tricks of the trade? According to the American Association of Family Practitioners (AAFP), and the American Association of Pediatrics (AAP), there are effective and ineffective ways to discipline your child. Reprimand incorrectly, and your efforts could backfire, bringing out the naughty in your child instead of the nice.

Positive Reinforcement

The following are disciplinary methods recognized by the distinguished associations mentioned above. Choose whether you believe the statement is "T" for true or "F" for false.

1. Positive reinforcement is effective on children of all ages. T or F?

2. Parents often make the mistake of giving a child more attention when they do something wrong than when they do something right. T or F?

3. Putting a gold star on a chart or a sticker on the child's shirt are forms of positive reinforcement. T or F?

4. Positive reinforcement doesn't have to involve a toy or physical prize; a smile or hug can be equally effective. T or F?

5. Positive reinforcement is most effective when done consistently and immediately after the desired behavior. T or F?

All of the above statements are true. Experts recommend that parents carefully choose their words so that they praise the action instead of the child. Saying "Good job!" applauds and encourages *doing* good, while "Good boy!" focuses the attention on simply *being* good. The experts also recommend praising a child frequently but to avoid celebrating a child's every action. Putting a toy away for example warrants a gold star on the forehead; playing with a toy does not. Overdo the high-fives and they become meaningless or expected at every occasion.

Time-Outs

Frequently used but infrequently done correctly, time-outs are a disciplinary technique that takes effort.

Test your time-out IQ by taking the quiz below:

1. Time-outs are most effective on children over six years old. T or F?

2. If a child knows a parent is serious about a time-out, they will stay put in the corner. T or F?

3. Discussing the reasons for the punishment during the time-out increases their effectiveness. T or F?

4. The worse the offense, the longer the time a child should spend in time-out. T or F?

5. Time-outs are best used when a child spills drinks, drops an object, or does other acts of clumsiness. T or F?

This popular disciplinary technique is far from fool-proof. Time-outs are most effective on children 18 months to six years old, making the first statement, and all the rest, false. You can be red-faced and steaming out the ears, pleading and still have to deal with a child that won't stay put (#2). Talking to a child when they're in exile negates the purpose of the punishment, (#3). And a child shouldn't spend more than one minute per year of age in time-out (four years old = four minutes time-out), or be penalized for normal childhood accidents such as wetting their pants or spilling the milk (# 4 and #5). Few parents are successful at their first attempts at time-outs, but with practice and tenacity, success will come.

Spanking and scolding

Over 90 percent of families admit that they have used spanking to discipline their child, despite the evidence of many drawbacks. Before making a decision on whether to swat or not, take the quiz below:

1. Too much scolding can encourage bad behavior because a child learns that's how he will get the most attention. T or F?

2. Scolding when used alone increases the chance that a child will ignore the requested good behavior. T or F?

3. Spanking is most commonly used on boys and by poor families. T or F?

4. Scolding is most effective on children under 18 months. T or F?

5. Studies show adults often harbor feelings of anger over being spanked as children. T or F?

All the statements above are true. Corporal punishment (spanking, shaking, or striking with belt or other object, such as a wooden spoon) will definitely cause a reaction in a child, and maybe immediate compliance, but doing so does not promote long-term good behavior. Parents are constantly being encouraged to find other ways of disciplining their children that aren't so damaging. Withholding treats or toys, implementing time-outs, or assigning an extra chore are all effective alternatives. Your pediatrician can also suggest programs focusing on ending the hand-to-the-backside habit.

Verbal Explanations/Rule Making

Good communications seems to be the magic pill to cure all social ills, but can it calm an unruly toddler? Take the quiz below to see if you know the right way to talk-the-talk:

1. Explaining drawbacks of bad behavior is best started while the child is still an infant. T or F?

2. It's important to explain to a child what rules were broken immediately, even if you're very angry. T or F?

3. Letting a child choose their punishment for breaking a rule undermines a parent's authority. T or F?

4. Repeat a rule over and over again, and your child will think it's nagging and tune you out. T or F?

5. Explaining the house rules is not as important as explaining the punishment that will be given if the rules are broken. T or F?

It's true that verbal explanations are a good discipline technique, but all of the statements above are false. Patiently explaining why it's not OK to throw food across the table is a waste of time on children under 18 months (#1), since they haven't reached the age of reason, and it can be downright frightening if you're so angry you look like a volcano ready to explode (#2). Involving your child with making and enforcing rules is a good idea since it allows him/her to feel responsible (#3), while repeating and explaining the benefits of the rules increases the chances that they will be followed (#4 and #5).

When and how will you apply these disciplinary techniques?

You watch a little boy steal a cookie off someone's plate, pull a cat's tail, kick over a game of building blocks, hit a sleeping baby, and then throw himself on the sofa to have the mother of all tantrums. You wish he belonged to someone else, but no, he's all yours. What demon has possessed the little boy with the angelic face that gave you such a heart-melting hug mere minutes ago? More importantly, what, if anything, will you do about it?

Using the information you've acquired above, choose which of the following technique you'll use on common childhood misbehaviors described below. If you think the offense doesn't deserve time in the penalty box, and can be dismissed, simply put an X in the corresponding spot. After making your choice, describe in detail how you'll carry out the punishment.

Punish or Pass?

PR = positive reinforcement TO= time-out VP= verbal punishment CP=corporal punishment VE= verbal explanation X = let it go.

What would you do if your child…

wouldn't stay in bed despite your orders and threats of punishment?   _____

refused to bathe or brush his teeth?   _____

played ball in the house or jumped on the furniture?   _____

drew on the walls or ruined a household item while playing?   _____

regularly had a fit at bedtime?   _____

took so long to complete simple tasks that they never got finished?   _____

refused to eat the food you prepared?   _____

repeatedly threw food on the floor during meal time (or gave his food to the dog under the table)?   _____

refused to eat anything except gummy candies for days?   _____

had the mother of all tantrums in a store?   _____

hit you while you were trying to discipline him?   _____

was driving you crazy by sassing back with "NO!" or "Shut up!" every time you made a request?   _____

screamed every time he didn't get his way?   _____

pointed and repeated "I want, I want" to everything in every store, making shopping extremely difficult?   _____

hit another child during playgroup?   _____

got hysterical and kept running to you over the slightest frustration?   _____

wet the bed?   _____

was running around your house naked in front of company?   _____

kept leaving his jacket or other items at the day care center or other location?   _____

blurted out an insensitive (and embarrassing) comment like "You smell funny" or "You're really fat" to a total stranger?   _____

played in the dirt and got filthy immediately after you've bathed and dressed him up in a new, clean outfit.   _____

made a mess in the kitchen and broke your favorite coffee mug while trying to serve himself juice without permission?   _____

denied eating the last piece of cake despite having a face full of frosting?   _____

hid candy under her shirt when you were grocery shopping?   _____

faked being sick or injured?   _____

Enforcing your rules and punishing bad behaviors is not an exact science with a one-size-fits-all solution. Parents are perpetually worried that their punishments don't fit their child's crimes. Effective disciplining involves a lot of trial and error, so don't become discouraged by the missteps. And, just when you think you've figured it all out, something will change in your child to start the crazy process all over again.

What will you do if you can't get your child to behave?

"I hope I don't get reported for this, but when they had tantrums in which counting to three or time-outs wouldn't help, I brought out the water spray bottle—yes, like training a dog, A quick squirt in the head usually snapped them right out of their attitude. A few times I had to use a whole bottle of water in the car. Yes, my back seat was soaked, but after a while, I just had to say 'I'm going to get the water bottle!' and they'd behave."

-Kathe, mother of 9- and 13-year-old sons

You see them on TV, or maybe you know a couple like them in real life. They are the parents who send out an SOS to a celebrity nanny to help them rein in their out-of-control children and rescue the family from a suburban version of *Lord of the Flies.*

What can you do to avoid the same predicament? Below are several common disciplinary scenarios. How you answer them will provide some clue as to whether you'll be unintentionally teaching your child to undermine your authority.

1. Would you fail to enforce a rule if it were broken while company was over to avoid causing a scene?

2. Could you see yourself being too tired after a long day to enforce the rules or follow up on a promised punishment?

3. If your child doesn't put away her toys as you asked, will you pick them up yourself rather than see the house messy?

4. If your child doesn't clean her room when asked, will you simply keep the door closed?

5. Will bedtime be at 7:30 unless there's a TV program on that your child enjoys watching?

6. Would it be OK to buy and share a hot pretzel from the mall food court, even though your rule is, "No snacking between meals?"

7. Will you postpone a punishment because it would interfere with a birthday party, soccer game, or family gathering?

8. Will you fail to enforce a time-out if your child wandered away from the designated time-out area?

9. Would you revoke or reduce a punishment if your child showed enough remorse?

10. If your child were grounded, could she still have friends over or play on the computer?

11. Will your child be able to hold on to a toy or take a book to the time-out corner?

12. If you gave your child permission to play with a friend but later remembered that she was grounded, would you simply drop the issue?

13. Would you reverse or lessen a punishment imposed by your partner?

14. Would you make a house rule or impose a punishment on your child and not tell your partner about it?

15. Would you apologize to your child for a punishment given by your partner or say something such as, "I would change things if I could?"

If you've answered "yes" to the majority of questions above, you might be setting yourself up to be a future member of the Disciplinarian Hall of Shame. According to the experts, lack of consistency and diligence when enforcing rules is the most common reason why parents lose the upper hand with their children. Without a doubt it's easier to give in to the screaming demon-child demanding a candy bar when you're at the checkout counter of a busy supermarket. But doing so leaves a clear message that tantrums work to get what you want. The more you give in, the more you'll reinforce this behavior.

Couples who don't appear united and have different rules and follow-through are perfect fodder for a child to exploit. Don't say you've never used the "Daddy (or Nanna) said it was OK" ploy when you were a child. Like the oxen in Aesop's fable, *The Four Oxen and the Lion*, parents must remember, "United we stand. Divided we fall."

Thankfully there's a tremendous amount of resources available online, through your healthcare provider, or from community groups that can help nip self-defeating habits in the bud. In many cases, the first step toward the successful disciplining of a child is to first discipline the parents.

CHAPTER 11

Special Parenting

"What do you mean Holland? I signed up for Italy!"

-Emily Perl Kingsley, from "Welcome to Holland"

Emily Pearl Kingsley, mother of a child with Down syndrome, wrote a famous piece describing how raising a disabled child was like being forced to land in one country when you've planned to visit another. Giving birth to twins (or other multiples), a child with impairments, or deciding to become a single parent is like having to vacation in a country that wasn't on your itinerary: It may not have been your original plan, but once there, you'll see unique events, visit beautiful places and meet wonderful people—all things you would have otherwise missed had you not been rerouted.

Finding out you'll be "parenting-plus" may seem a little daunting, Raising a child is special in its own right, but some parents have a few more eggs in their baskets to contend with. But as any parent who has held the job before you would confirm, it comes with tremendously rewarding emotional perks that last a lifetime.

What unique situations should you expect as a parent of multiples?

"When raising multiples extra help is mandatory, it's definitely all hands on deck. Get your mother, sister, or hire help if you can. Go to a relative's house if possible. You need to call in the troops. Next, join a twins club. I joined before I delivered, which was great. I got to hear birth stories which were helpful, and the members can really help you with resources. Even if you already had a child, you'll need the extra stroller, car seat, and everything else. It's also nice to have the camaraderie with other parents who are in the same boat. When our twins got older, we even formed an identical twin soccer league."

-Lois, mother to a 22-year-old son and 20-year-old twin girls

The Mayans believed twins were a blessing; so did the ancient Romans, as long as both were boys. Bearing twins holds special meaning in almost all cultures. For parents, it usually means double the work, yet undoubtedly double the love, too. Similar but separate, twins are a bonus pack of love—double the giggles, double the hugs. Because multiple share so many things, they are naturals at "playing well with others" and often teach *parents* how to compromise.

If you find you'll be carrying a trio (or more!) of heartbeats, prepare yourself for the following situations unique to parents of multiples by answering the next set of questions.

1. Will you welcome or downplay the extra attention your multiples get?

2. How will you handle any jealous feelings from other moms about the extra attention your multiples may receive?

3. Will you be more inclined to hire a nanny or to become a SAHP if you find out you'll be delivering multiples?

4. Will you insist your multiples dress alike, even if they don't want to?

5. Will you insist they dress differently to reinforce that they are individuals?

6. What will you do if your multiples insisted on doing everything together and exactly alike?

7. Will you make big changes in how you manage your family's finances knowing multiples are on their way?

8. Will you join a twins or multiples support group or social club?

9. Will you be open to having your multiples participate in non-invasive (questionnaires, motor skills tests, etc.) scientific research on twins?

10. Will you expect both to reach milestones (walking, talking, potty training, etc.) at the same time? What (if anything) will you do if one lags behind the other?

11. What (if anything) will you say if people labeled one of your multiples the "pretty twin" or the "smart twin?"

12. Do you think it's important to make sure you're giving each multiple individual time and attention? If so, how will this be achieved?

13. What will you do if your multiples start swapping places in school and perform other lighthearted twin pranks?

14. If you can't tell which one of your multiples was the instigator of a prank, would you punish both?

15. What would you do if your twins' personalities were as different as night and day and they bickered constantly?

As the average age for a first-time pregnancy ticks up, so does the incidence of pregnancies carrying multiples. Women who conceive after 25 years of age have higher levels of the hormones that increase the chance of becoming pregnant with twins or triplets. Medical advances also have a hand in swelling the numbers— women undergoing fertility regiments such as in vitro fertilization or taking fertility drugs to help conceive are more likely to conceive multiples.

How should you prepare for parenting a special needs child?

"If I could have parents choose which disability their child would have, it would be Down syndrome. These children are so giving, so loving; my (afflicted) son is the heart of our family. It really is a blessing, and the people I've met because of my son are amazing. I would never have made the friendships I have if it were not for his condition."

-Donnell, mother to a 16-year-old son

and a 12-year-old son with Down syndrome

The increased prevalence of Autism Spectrum Disorder (ASD), Trisomy 21 (Down syndrome), and severe food allergies in children have earned all of these conditions added attention in society. If these increasing numbers create concerns that your soon-to-be-born child could contribute to the trend, keep in mind that 97 percent of all babies are born *without* birth defects, and the vast majority of children will not show signs of developmental disabilities.

If you discover your child will likely be born with a medical condition, there is plenty of good news. The science and social programs offering support and treatment for many childhood disabilities get better by the day. The questions below will help if you find yourself preparing to be parents to a child that requires special attention.

What are some considerations when becoming a parent to a child with special needs?

1. Will you contact agencies and organizations that help parents with special needs children to ask for aid and support?
2. Will you be willing to move to an area that offers more programs and better medical care for children with special needs?
3. Will you only agree to tests your doctor suggests that address an immediate illness, or will you be open to experimental treatments or using untested methods to treat or study your child's condition?
4. Will you cut your special needs child slack when they misbehave?
5. Will you be adamant to make sure your special needs child is part of your family, not the center of your family?
6. How insistent and dedicated will you be to "mainstreaming" your child?
7. Do you know your state's laws regarding your child's right to an education and the mandates your local school must follow?
8. How will you handle ignorant assumptions and comments that your child's physical or emotional disabilities are due to your poor parenting?
9. How will you modify your finances and insurance policies to have the means to provide necessary medical care?
10. What conditions might make you feel that your child would be better off living in assisted housing (mental/physical institution)?

There's no denying that having a child with a severe birth or developmental defect is challenging, but there are rewards. Parents raising a child with special needs will confess that it forced them to do extraordinary feats of personal fortitude and emotional strength that they otherwise wouldn't have attempted, let alone accomplish, had their child been born without ailments.

With this strength comes support. Of all the ways technology has improved our lives, the ability for parents to reach out and obtain information from the medical community or to network with kindred souls has been one of its greatest contributions.

What are considerations when raising a child as an unmarried couple?

Contrary to popular opinion, marriage is more than just a piece of paper. It's a fast pass to all sorts of legal privileges between you, your child, and your partner. You both may have promised each other that you'll raise your child as a loving, committed couple, but until you've signed on the dotted line (of a marriage certificate or paternity agreement), in the eyes of the law, you're a single parent family. If you'll be raising a child as an unmarried couple there are legal and logistical concerns you'll need to address to protect your rights and the best interests of your baby.*

1. Does your state require a signed affidavit establishing paternity before allowing an unmarried father to sign the birth certificate or have any legal parental rights?

2. If your baby's father does not file an affidavit establishing paternity, could your child be denied any of the father's Social Security survivor benefits or insurance policy survivor payouts?

3. If your partner is not established as a legal parent, could he/she lose custody of your child should you (the legal parent) die or become disabled?

4. If your partner has not filed a court custody arrangement, could the baby's mother remarry and have her new husband adopt your child without your consent?

5. Could your child be denied enrollment in a church parish, private club, or other private program because of your marital status?

6. If filing separate tax returns, who will claim your child as a dependent?

7. If you lose your health benefits due to unemployment, will you be unable to gain coverage for your child through your partner's policy?

8. If your partner was previously married, will he/she amend Social Security files so your child can also receive benefits?

9. Does your state allow same-sex partners to sign a child's birth certificate?

10. If your state does not allow same-sex parenting, what legal protections do you have to ensure shared custody and protection under the law?

*Since we've touched upon some legal issues, here's the mandatory disclaimer: the above quiz and any other information contained in this book should not be considered legal counsel. Contact an attorney if you have any questions or need information regarding custodial rights and other family law matters.

What steps can you take to successfully raise a child by yourself?

Raising a child solo can be unnerving, but if you find comfort in numbers, the following should make you feel cozy: The latest U.S. Government reports 41 percent of births are to single women, and in California there's been a 20 percent increase in the number of single women seeking sperm donations from the California Cryobank (the nation's largest sperm bank). In other words, if you've chosen to raise a child by yourself, you're definitely not alone.

Being part of a large group doesn't necessarily mean you're safe from feeling isolated or unsupported. Single parents consistently list finances, time, alienation, and inadequacy as their top concerns. If you're stressing over the same list, ask yourself the questions below to see if you're addressing these concerns in the best possible manner and are willing to do what's necessary to avoid these sandpits of single parenthood.

If you're concerned about how you're going to make ends meet with only one income...

1. have you explored all the social programs offering financial aid for single parents?

2. have you thought of going back to school to increase your earning potential?

3. will you talk to your employer about increasing your responsibilities, hours, and pay?

4. are you taking serious steps to create a financial plan, or are you simply hoping your money matters will work themselves out somehow?

5. will you refuse to let guilt, pity, or insecurities cause you to buy more gifts, toys, and clothes for your child than she needs or than you can afford?

Solo parenting does not guarantee a life of poverty. There's plenty of financial assistance for single parents, literally at your fingertips. A few keystrokes on your phone or computer and a plethora of sites and organizations will pop up on your screen announcing tips, services, and communities eager to help you make ends meet.

If you're worried about not being up to the challenge of raising a child alone...

1. are you willing to accept that being a parent means you'll have both good and bad days, with a few mega mistakes thrown in every now and then?

2. will you build up the courage to cut out people, pets, or activities that take up valuable time and add to your stress load?

3. will you have your child help you do housework (laundry, dishwashing, yard work) as soon as they're able?

4. will refuse to run yourself ragged just to prove that you can do it all yourself?

5. will you continuously search for parenting tips and inspiration from experts who have positive experiences with solo parenting?

When all the responsibilities fall on your shoulders, it's necessary to lighten the load or be crushed. Don't want to go crazy commuting? Only sign up your child for one play group or none, and don't sign up to take cupcakes to every school party when you barely have enough time to make dinner. The most powerful word in your vocabulary will be "No." Learn to use it when being sucked dry by needy adults or when you're about to beat yourself up for not being involved in every school or children's program in your neighborhood. The lesson parents learn very quickly is that doing everything poorly is never as good as choosing to do fewer things well.

If you're worried about being alienated or unsupported...

1. will you extend an olive branch to those who disapprove of you becoming a single parent and work on creating a civil relationship?

2. will you follow blogs or participate in parenting forums to broaden your support group- even if it's only online?

3. will you avoid using your child as an excuse for not going out and meeting people or being open to a romantic relationship?

4. will you adopt the belief that for every friendship you lose by becoming a parent, two new ones can take its place?

5. will you organize a babysitting co-op with other parents to expand your social circle?

If the number of parenting blogs is any indication, solo parents love talking to other solos and creating social networks, so there's no excuse for not making new friends. If your current social contacts don't offer comfort or encourage your solo parenting plight, find new ones. Don't waste your time looking for their approval. Your role as a parent is to raise a healthy, happy child, not to please your friends. Stick with people who will help not hinder your ability to accomplish this goal. It may sound harsh and hard to do, but it's not impossible.

If you're worried about keeping your child away from any baby-daddy/
mama drama...

1. will you and the baby's father be negotiating a custody or visitation
   agreement with an attorney before your baby is born?
2. even if you were angry at your ex, will you always try to present him/her
   in a positive light for the sake of your child?
3. will you avoid discussing your problems with your ex and his/her family
   in front of your child?
4. will you have a rule to never get in a loud fight with your ex in front of
   your child?
5. are you adamant about never using your child as a pawn to get back at
   your ex no matter how big of a jerk he or she may have been?

Like it or not you, your child, and your ex have a life-long connection that can't
be severed. You may cringe at the sound of your baby daddy's name, but his blood
runs through your child's veins, as does yours. Criticize your child's father, and
you're putting down a part within your own child. This is why it's so important
to do everything possible to maintain a civil relationship with your ex, no matter
how terribly he treated you. Your child will have a natural desire to love his father
and his mother. You should consider that feeling sacred and do everything in your
power to promote a sense of love and respect between the three of you. Even if
your relationship is strained, find some way to agree on parenting ground rules.
As Luisa, single mother of a 13-year-old explains, "I told my daughter's dad that
we had to be on the same page when disciplining our daughter. We can't show that
one is weak and the other is strong, because she will use that against us."

FINAL THOUGHTS

Expecting a baby is a time filled with wonder, speculation, excitement, and yes, anxiety. What will labor feel like exactly? Will my child be born healthy? Will I be a good parent?" However, instead of losing sleep over the unknown, enjoy dreaming about the possibilities. From the moment of conception, your child exists– a unique creation, whose unequalled characteristics will reveal themselves, slowly, day-by-day as her parents watch with awe.

Christy, the mother of three sons, remembers observing her then-young children with fascination, wondering how their personalities would take shape with time and age. Now that her sons have grown into wonderful young adults, she sees how each son's individual personality and passions came to fruition in their lives. Her eldest son, who liked to hike outdoors, became a geologist. The son who loved to read became a teacher. "I learned quickly that kids have innate abilities that have nothing to do with parenting skills," she confessed.

Which brings to mind an analogy: Imagine that parents are similar to a dam, the type that's a huge marvel of modern engineering. The roaring river is their child, en route to its destiny. If the dam completely stops the flow of the water, it will never fulfill its purpose. Let the water flow unrestricted and unguided, and its potential is wasted. If the dam correctly handles the force of the river—not by changing it, but by managing and guiding its natural flow—its water can bring life to arid land, and light to millions.

The joys of parenthood are unmatched, as are the tough times. But many things in life are difficult. Some of these challenges we embrace because they allow us to grow and show—or discover—that there's a superman or woman within us. Becoming a parent forces you to put on that superhero cape and fight the righteous fight. To borrow a phrase made famous by the Peace Corps, parenting will be "The toughest job you'll ever love."

ABOUT THE AUTHOR

Monica Mendez Leahy has been helping couples prepare for life changing milestones for over twenty years, and has married over 100 couples as a Deputy Commissioner of Civil Marriages for the County of Los Angeles. She hosts a series of popular workshops for couples in the Los Angeles area and provides private classes to engaged and newlywed couples both in person, and online.

Her advice on relationships is frequently sought after and has been featured in various TV and radio programs in addition to articles in the *Ladies Home Journal,* the *Wall Street Journal* and other prominent national publications. She has served on panels along with other notable authors such as John Gray, of *Venus and Mars* fame and Harville Hendrix. Couples can also seek her advice through her articles, and at **www.1001questionstoask.com.**

.

Made in the USA
Coppell, TX
21 November 2020